IVF

Infertility and IVF

Facts and Feelings from Patients' Perspectives

Jo Benson and
Dawn Robinson-Walsh

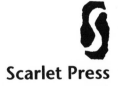

Scarlet Press

Published by Scarlet Press 1998
5 Montague Road, London E8 2HN

British Library Cataloguing-in-Publication Data
A catalogue record for this book is available
from the British Library

ISBN 1 85727 093 2 pb

Designed and produced for Scarlet Press by
Chase Production Services, Chadlington, OX7 3LN
Typeset from the authors' disk by
Stanford Desktop Publishing Services, Northampton
Printed in the EC by J.W. Arrowsmith, Bristol

To Christine and Wendy, may the babies you desperately want be forthcoming soon; to Cheryl and Andrew, with congratulations; and to Marcia who is a very 'special lady'.

Contents

Acknowledgements

The authors would like to offer thanks to the many contributors who helped with the case studies for this book. Their frankness and honesty in discussing such a painful subject is testimony to their feeling that there is a real need for a book offering patients' perspectives on infertility and its treatment. Thanks also to Clare Brown, Executive Director of Child, who freely offered her help and support, both in providing information and in reading the completed text. Finally, our thanks to Derek Tuffnell, Consultant Obstetrician and Gynaecologist at Bradford Royal Infirmary whose help was so useful and so willingly given.

1 What is the problem?

'Go forth and multiply ...'

In 1996 a Sunday supplement led with the shocking headline question: 'Is infertility a new threat to humanity?' It was highlighting the fact that the moment of natural conception is an increasingly rare event, with a growing number of couples having to resort to unpleasant and costly medical or surgical treatments. It is believed that one in six couples have trouble conceiving. In a third of cases this is due to sperm problems, in another third to female problems and in the final third to joint problems relating to both partners. Fertility expert Professor Lord Robert Winston estimates that there are 600,000 British couples suffering infertility for a variety of reasons, all of which deserve proper diagnosis before treatment can begin. Studies in the UK of the prevalence of infertility are difficult to correlate because of the widely different definitions, population studies and methods of research that they use. The three latest population-based studies have found infertility rates within the UK to be 13.7 per cent, 24.2 per cent and 15.2 per cent, respectively. It is generally concluded, and confirmed throughout the western world, that the lifetime prevalence of infertility varies from 13.7 per cent to 24 per cent, with the majority of studies agreeing on an overall rate of 15 per cent. It is thus, a problem on a huge scale, which has to be tackled with finite resources, using diagnostic techniques that are time-consuming and in many cases limited in effect.

For couples relying on the National Health Service there are a whole series of wider problems and issues to be tackled before the micro level of individual lives and hopes is reached. There are many theories as to why infertility appears to be a problem of the 1990s. New research into reproductive technology is badly needed. Stonehouse, for example, raises the point that research into problems with sperm is a relatively new area, because fertility problems have historically been connected with women rather than men.[1] Yet the funding of university departments undertaking such research is being cut; for instance, Sheffield University used to work in close liaison with the Jessop Hospital, but that hospital closed in 1996. Is infertility research funding an easy target because infertility and the desire for a baby are still generally perceived as a woman's issue? Women's medicine and midwifery have been traditionally underfunded, perhaps because the decision-makers – both scientific and political – have tended to be men.

Infertility offers emotional pain and a good deal of anguish for affected couples, as people grapple to come to terms with the simple fact that we are not always in control of our bodies despite various attempts to achieve some degree of control. To some extent we have wanted (and had) some control through advances in (female oral) contraceptive techniques, and now it appears that a price is being paid for this by some. Women have used technology (often the contraceptive pill, the coil (IUD), and, more recently, injectables such as depo-provera and implants, which either disturb hormone production and levels within the body or – in the case of the coil – is linked with uterine infections) to avoid pregnancy; so far, little has been done to develop similar effective male contraceptives. In the belief that we can delay our natural fertility, the whole issue of reproduction is left until potential parents are far older than the age that is now recognised as biologically helpful. As the ageing process continues without mercy, the biological clock starts ticking and there is very little time to tackle the problem. It seems we cannot 'have it all', despite the promises of the women's magazines of the 1970s. Late-age pregnancy can be problematic in terms of poorer egg quality, a lower conception rate, and greater risk of ectopic pregnancies, miscarriages and lengthier deliveries. It also means that the woman has had more time to develop sexually transmitted diseases (often unknowingly) or to have had a therapeutic abortion. As Professor Roger Gosden of Leeds University asserts, 'Deferring fertility is a gamble.'

Early sexual activity is also an unquantifiable aspect of today's fertility problems. The 'freedoms' associated with the pill during the 1960s, 70s and 80s, including the abandoning of the old (but now deemed useful) barrier methods of contraception such as male condoms, have meant that young women are more likely to develop sexually transmitted infections. The condom not only acted as a barrier to sperm but also helped to protect women and men from a number of infections.

There has certainly been a tendency, too, to ignore early symptoms of 'menstrual' problems in women such as the onset of endometriosis, a condition which can lead to great heartache later and is still not fully understood. Many contributors to this book have reported that as teenagers they experienced excruciating pain around the time of their periods – something which is simply not normal and should be investigated – but their concerns were brushed aside, only for the women to discover later the damage done to their reproductive systems. Likewise, it is now recognised that the infection chlamydia may play a major part in fertility problems, yet still there is no nationwide screening process for this common infection, which is often symptomless as it wreaks silent damage upon its victims.

The need to have babies

Why the imperative to have a family? In a questionnaire issued to a number of couples, the replies received were generally similar (completed by women) and linked to societal expectations as much as to any biological imperative:

> Vanessa: 'It's a natural progression in a loving relationship; I love and get on well with children and would like to complete our family unit.'
>
> Lena: 'Children are part of the meaning of life and it is also a biological need to have children.'
>
> Helen: 'Ever since I can remember, I had always wanted to be a Mummy; I felt very maternal and this became even worse when my brother had a family.'
>
> Jean: 'A normal, natural thing to do. There are many social pressures – as a childless couple we often get left out of things; it would make my life more complete.'
>
> Imogen: 'Having children is expected of you; it feels as if something is missing without; you are not complete; it is for your own fulfilment.'

While most people questioned talked of fulfilment and biological need, a good proportion also recognised that it is societal pressure to conform to the perceived norm of the family unit which plays a huge part in developing feelings of loss, non-belonging and being 'different' among those who have no children. This is despite the fact that the Cornflake-packet family structure with husband, wife and 2.2 children barely exists in reality. The image of the happy family remains a strong pull.

There is of course a gender aspect to the question of fertility, with childless women allegedly feeling the isolation and sense of failure much more keenly than men even though infertility affects men and women in approximately equal numbers, but the whole stereotype of a typically infertile couple needs addressing too. Rose states that the generally accepted stereotype is that of a childless couple, desperately anguished by their shared condition, but in these days of serial monogamy this is often not the case.[2] She cites the story of Jan Brennan, a successful participant in the Australian Monash In vitro fertilisation (IVF) programme in 1982. Her partner Les Brennan was already married when she met him, and the father of six children whom he had left behind. At the time, Jan was unlikely to have received IVF had she been a single woman wanting a baby, or a partner in a lesbian relationship. She needed a male partner to legitimate her desire in the eyes of the obstetricians.

Among people interviewed for this book, it has certainly seemed that a baby is more of an issue for the female partner in a relationship. But it also has to be said that while many couples desperately would like to have children, there are others who deal with the issue differently – some, for example, investigate the options open to them in their quest to have a child and decide that the whole invasive process of IVF is not for them. This is currently an issue with at least one contributor to this book, who has undergone numerous tests, is on the verge of reaching the end of her local NHS IVF waiting list and is having serious second thoughts about the whole procedure.

For many people, however, infertility is not something which can be assessed rationally; it is an agonising emotional weight:

> Imogen: 'I felt a failure; my husband feels that there is life without children though he would also like to have them.'
> Jean: 'I grew very depressed, I lost weight, my life fell apart. I still cannot accept it, but my husband then denied that he had wanted children because he felt anger that he couldn't produce offspring; i.e. "be a man".'

Vanessa: 'Disbelief; I still don't believe that I will never have children. My husband feels similarly, but he is more concerned about me; he has the attitude of "if it's meant to be, it'll happen".'

Lena: 'I was very depressed; my husband thought that we could either learn to live without children or adopt them.'

Helen: 'We both felt complete and utter devastation.'

Male infertility is becoming an increasingly important and talked-about issue, although debate is still very muted compared with female infertility. The charity Foresight (the Association for the Promotion of Preconceptual Care)[3] claims that there is very little research available which is directly concerned with male infertility. Stonehouse comments that sperm counts have reduced over the past years by 50 per cent, according to figures in Britain, the USA and Sweden.[4] This seems to be a worldwide problem. Sperm samples have also included high numbers of sperm incapacitated in some way, such as having a deformed head or tail, or little motility. Sperm are the smallest body cells and are thought to be vulnerable to pollutants, especially manmade oestrogens in water. Rates of testicular cancer have also risen, while the number of boys with undescended testicles has doubled in 30 years. Coburn, Peterson Myers and Dumanoski speculate on the threat to reproduction posed by manmade chemicals, citing the world decline in human sperm count and the rise in testicular cancer as examples of humans being used as part of an unregulated global experiment[5] – an idea seized upon by the growing organic movement, concerned by the poor information and knowledge that people have about the effects of agrochemicals, irradiation and genetic engineering to produce cheap food.

Foresight is convinced that male infertility – whether this involves low sperm count, poor motility, malformations, clumping (sperm adhering together) or no sperm at all – is linked to health problems which may often be corrected by changes to diet and habits, such as giving up alcohol and tobacco. Genito-urinary infections are also a source of problems, as are vitamin and mineral deficiencies. Preconceptual care is an issue which is often ignored but should be the first port of non-invasive investigation. To continue the argument concerning environmental hazards to male fertility, Foresight lists the following substances as known or suspected to be harmful to male reproductive health: lead, dibromochloropropane, or DBCP (a now banned soil fumigant), ionising and non-ionising radiation, anaesthetic gases, vinyl chloride (used in the manufacture of plastics), the pesticide kepone, heat stress, carbon disulphide (used in the manufacture of viscose rayon), oestrogen (used in manufacturing oral contraceptives), methylene chloride (used as a solvent) and ethylene bromide, or EDB (used in leaded petrol). Foresight also provides a comprehensive list of other industrial reproductive hazards.

Foresight is part of a growing group of people who are concerned about increasing medical and surgical interventions in fertility when the causes of infertility may well be environmental or a product of poor nutrition – an assessment that is hotly debated by people who are not so convinced but one that is surely worth investigating by couples in the throes of fertility problems, at least as something positive to be doing while awaiting IVF. The charity offers screening for nutritional deficiencies but also checking to detect ovulation, assessment of the hormonal balance necessary for conception, semen analysis, checking of the uterus and fallopian tubes and checking the friendliness of vaginal mucus to sperm. Testing differs from conventional medicine in that it avoids intervention as much as possible; for example, the evaluation of the uterus and fallopian tubes is done by SHG (sonohysterogram) instead of hysterosalpingogram (HSG), which uses X-ray, or laparoscopy, which involves use of a general anaesthetic.

It is easy to dismiss such theories and alternative challenges to conventional wisdom on infertility as unscientific or unrealistic, but the evidence is interesting. The Foresight Preconception Research Study of 1990–2 involved 367 couples, of whom 136 females and 94 males had reported a previous history of reproductive problems concerning infertility. Some cases involved both partners, so 204 couples had an infertility problem. After the completion of questionnaires and analyses/treatments, a follow-up in 1993 revealed that 175 healthy children had been conceived, all of whom were carried to term and were perfectly healthy. Of the couples, 46 had reported previous failed IVF treatments on between one and four occasions. Following the programme, 30 women in this group had become pregnant, resulting in 30 normal deliveries of single, healthy babies.

The popular response is often to assume that people shouldn't get too upset when pregnancy doesn't happen. Many people (often those with children) are of the opinion that if it is meant to happen, it will happen. But history shows that fertility has always been an issue, and that couples have undergone extraordinary rituals to achieve pregnancy. Taking examples from the sixteenth century, Jacques Gélis notes that royal family members would visit holy shrines and countrywomen would make symbols of fertility, offer grain to a newlywed woman, or kill a chicken before a wedding ceremony to make fertility certain, so feared was barrenness and sterility.[6] Gélis states that not only did the infertile follow fertility rites, but so did anyone embarking on a relationship until fertility was ascertained by the achievement of a pregnancy. The unmarried woman at this time (not the bachelor) was cut off from the social fabric; woman's status derived from husband and children, without them she would be marginalised. Remnants of this set of beliefs and attitudes seem to remain today, making the reproductive process of vital importance, especially to women.

The birth of IVF

Reproductive technology has so far, then, mainly focused on women. The history of infertility treatment for women has shown that such treatments have often been little more than scientific and medical experimentation. Take the event seen as the origin of successful IVF: the birth of Lesley Brown's daughter Louise in 1978, which brought the whole issue of IVF to people's attention. Research was going on well before then, using human guinea pigs. Prior to the dramatic medical breakthrough by the pioneers, Robert Edwards and Patrick Steptoe, couples suffering from infertility had little hope of satisfactory treatment. Virtually all investigation centred on the woman, for example (with sperm count rarely being checked), and then mainly consisted of laparotomy (later laparoscopy, which was less traumatic and offered the same results) and a D&C after the usual look through the patient's history. If a patient, like the mother of Louise Brown, had no fallopian tubes or they were blocked, then adoption was probably the only path open to her if she wanted children. So, experimental though it was, 'breakthrough' is not too dramatic a description of the day when Steptoe secured an egg from the ovary of Lesley Brown and Edwards managed to fertilise the egg in the laboratory using her husband's sperm. Using a microscope, Edwards was able to watch the embryo divide into cells and Steptoe managed to replace the egg in Lesley Brown's womb. Science and medicine combined to achieve conception. Louise arrived nine months later on 26 July, delivered by Caesarean section. It all sounded so easy, but IVF today still has a high failure rate. The birth of Louise Brown was the result of ten years of persevering research and some degree of trial and error, with the goal of bringing hope to infertile couples. The result was a triumph of medicine linked with science but, according to many, Lesley Brown was the (albeit willing) object of experimentation, although no one would deny a person that choice. However, cynicism abounds and motivation in such cases is always questioned; as newspaper rights to the story at the time were reportedly sold for £300,000, the experiment was a success in more ways than one and set a base for the number of questions of ethics which have been raised about such treatments ever since.

Current discussion concerning the disposal of frozen embryos is a further development in the opposition to IVF which has always existed. In their book *A Matter of Life*, Steptoe and Edwards describe in detail the opposition they encountered from religious groups, official sources, scientists and the medical profession. Indeed, the doctor and scientist were unwavering in their belief that cells taken from embryos should be used to alleviate disorders in people – to them the embryo was a collection of cells, not a foetus in recognisable human shape. That said, towards the end of their book they mention the need to guard against abuses, such as cloning (now a very real issue following the cloning of Dolly the sheep in 1997) and other forms of manipulation found within genetic engineering. In the quest for a child, the ethical questions probably do not worry would-be parents at the time of the treatment; later, they can become an issue.

One woman interviewed was at the stage of wondering what to do with her frozen embryos that were due to be destroyed; she clearly felt that it had become a difficult ethical issue for her. She felt that as biological mother she was in the difficult position of not wanting more children but feeling responsible for her potential babies. Unlike Messrs Steptoe and Edwards, she saw her embryos as effectively babies; conversely, her husband did not feel the same attachment and, knowing of the agonies of infertility felt it was selfish not to donate them for use by other childless couples or for research.

Ann Oakley raises the point that reproductive technology such as IVF has enabled men to achieve what they have always wanted – certainty and proof of fatherhood.[7] The father can be assured that it is his sperm being used in the fertilisation process – something that no man in unassisted conception can be certain of. Certainly, it appears that the male has a fairly minor role to play in the procedure but may secure great rewards if it is successful. This feminist argument may not appeal to many, but an alternative, unrelated point may strike a chord with the majority – IVF, like abortion, is a lottery; its availability depends on where you live and what medical help you have access to. IVF is provided for some at a cost to many because it uses funds which could be channelled into primary preventative health care aimed at eliminating the major causes of infertility for a greater number of sufferers; such a utilitarian argument is hard to fault unless you are infertile and stuck on a waiting list for IVF or, worse, denied treatment because of where you live and the problems of funding treatment. This is covered more fully in chapter 7.

Technology, then, has improved since the days of Steptoe and Edwards, but access to that technology is still under question. The nationwide average pregnancy rate (not birth rate) per cycle was 14.2 per cent in 1996. A patient's place of residence and medical links with specialist hospitals play a part in the chances of success, as does the willingness (or ability) of GPs to fund expensive drug treatments prior to surgery. However, despite the difficulties which have since come to light, the pioneers of infertility treatment, those women prepared to try IVF before it was established as a respected technique, were a very special group – as the interview with Marcia makes clear. Marcia was in her second marriage and had received ten years' worth of 'normal' infertility treatment in Oldham. She was a patient of Patrick Steptoe.

Marcia
He suggested I was put with his 'special ladies'. His team tested my husband's sperm; there was no problem with that. I was given 96 tablets and four injections per month to stimulate my egg production after a laparoscopy couldn't find anything wrong with me.

Mr Steptoe was a very fatherly man, patient and understanding. He was aware of the mental pain that infertile women suffered, and was sympathetic. He was wonderful. Looking back, it seems that being a pioneer was my job. We offered ourselves, we ladies, hoping it might work for one of us. I was in a group of six. He just said that he was going to try something different with us. Slowly, it dawned on me what he was saying – he was a very unassuming man. I was excited, but felt very safe; I knew he wouldn't do anything to harm me; I had absolute confidence and trust. It was another chance of getting a baby. I was a bit bothered about what would happen, and we were given very little information – I didn't ask; you didn't in those days. I was rather in awe of him; he was charismatic.

Marcia was given tablets to take every month – she didn't know what they were for. She also had to save all her urine:

I had to take a container everywhere – work, shopping – and dropped it off each day at the cottage hospital. I don't know what they did with it. Mr Steptoe sent for me three days before I went into hospital – I had to take three tablets, and I felt very sick. Then there was a phone call one night to tell me to go in – my bag was always ready. I had lots of blood tests. The technician who was taking blood was very rough – he wiggled the needle in the vein. It upset me and I fainted and threatened to tell Mr Steptoe. I fainted again when Mr Steptoe walked into the room. I woke up in a bed in a tiny ward. When I came round, Mr Steptoe was stroking my hair. He said, 'What these girlies will do to have babies.' When I stirred, he moved away and was back to normal.

I went to theatre and they took two eggs from me. My husband gave a sperm sample. Robert Edwards was there. Then my legs were put in stirrups and the fertilised eggs were put back inside with a catheter-type thing. It was physically uncomfortable. I had to stay for 24 hours with my legs slightly raised. The timing was very important.

Two weeks later, I had my period. I was devastated, crying and crying. Mr Steptoe said: 'I'll try again.' I needed time to pull myself together. We knew he was on the brink of success and it could be any one of us. He was desperately short of funding – people accused him of playing god, so things had to be kept quiet. We were in a hospital with other people around who were dying – it was quite traumatic and we were trying to keep quiet. The nursing staff weren't nice, but on the whole Mr Steptoe's special team looked after us. You weren't made to feel welcome.

When I heard about the Louise Brown success I was so pleased he'd done it but wished it could have been me as well. He then moved to Bourn Hall, Cambridge. By then I was nearly 40 and we let it go as I had promised my husband I would.

I later discovered there was nothing on my notes regarding my IVF with Mr Steptoe – he was considered a law unto himself and he kept the notes he took privately. There were no records – this is typical; he was protective of us and didn't want anyone to know about it. I had no regrets – I'd have regretted it if I hadn't tried.

These days, no one ever mentions the pioneers – they never talk about those who made it possible for others. People maligned Steptoe because of ignorance and lack of knowledge. Dr Edwards was also very nice – I wrote to him when Mr Steptoe died. Steptoe himself called us his 'special ladies'. You have to have a certain percentage of women who'll have a go, and I have a bit of pride that I did something for society. It is a nice feeling to know I contributed something, and I can't speak too highly of the doctors.

Marcia is right that the pioneers of infertility treatment are never mentioned, but that may be because of the secrecy affecting the research at the time. In truth, most people undergoing fertility treatment will probably never have thought about those who must have been first to try it. Despite Marcia's unstinting praise for Mr Steptoe, it is alarming today to realise that so little information was given to women prepared to try experimental treatment – the process sounded very cloak and dagger because of the risks of going public, but Marcia was a woman desperate for a baby who was prepared to be guided by the opinion of a doctor she trusted. Maybe today, with a refinement in technique, Marcia would have been an IVF success story. Talking about it now still brings her an emotional fullness which is impossible for anyone who hasn't been in the situation to empathise with fully. She was also a patient in days when even husband and wife were unlikely to discuss the issues at a deep level, and where a doctor's word would be accepted unquestioningly. Arguably, people today are more willing to challenge medical practitioners and certainly much more information is given prior to IVF treatment. In its literature, the HFEA (Human Fertilisation and Embryology Authority) encourages patients to ask questions and even offers examples of what these might be.

What is IVF?

Before any couple reaches the IVF stage, they are likely to have been trying for a baby for at least two years (less time in the case of older couples). The first port of call is the GP, who will usually arrange for tests to try to ascertain why conception has not been achieved. Before undergoing IVF, you are likely to be counselled about your reasons for wanting treatment and the causes of your fertility problem. The welfare of the child should also be considered, but what constitutes this is contentious. For example, in the 1996 BBC 1 television series *Making Babies*, Professor Lord Robert Winston's staff at Hammersmith Hospital were highly divided on this issue in a case where an HIV positive woman wanted to undergo IVF treatment. Professor Winston felt that it was not the medical profession's role to make qualitative social judgements, but many of his team clearly felt very uneasy over this ethical issue and a number of meetings were held to discuss it.

You may have blood tests, and tests to show that your eggs and sperm are not faulty. You will also be asked to give your consent on three issues: consent to the use and storage of your eggs and sperm and of any embryos produced (you may vary or withdraw this consent later, unless an embryo has already been used in treatment or for research); consent to your fertility treatment itself, such as egg retrieval and transfer of embryos; and consent to disclosure of identifying information, for example to your GP.

If you disclose to people that you are undergoing IVF treatment, it is worth being prepared for some negative reactions. Zipper and Sevenhuijsen note that women are considered egoistic if they want children but also if they don't[8] – a view which has been reinforced by our contributors. Women who become pregnant easily are 'normal', those who don't are labelled 'fanatical' and those who don't want to are not 'real women' in the eyes of society – you are damned if you do and damned if you don't. One woman who decided to be sterilised before she was 30 years old because she had decided she did not want children, and had suffered gynaecological problems which would undoubtedly make the process very difficult if she did, was viewed as 'over the top' by many of her peers, although some thought her 'brave' and one (male) felt that her decision was on the basis of post hoc rationalisation.

In society's eyes, however irrational or unjust it may seem, infertility treatment appears to be seen as acceptable for a very specific group of people. The Warnock Committee itself approved of IVF and artificial insemination as techniques for treating involuntarily infertile heterosexual couples in stable relationships. Surrogacy was disapproved of because of commercialism, but also as a signal of abhorrence and condemnation that a woman could give away her child, especially if this was a rational, conscious act.

Successes and stresses of IVF treatment

Since the birth of Louise Brown, 70 clinics have been set up in the UK to offer IVF treatment of varying degrees, all monitored by the HFEA, which provides a helpful booklet detailing treatments available and comparative success rates (see p. 149). IVF is mainly used where the woman in a partnership suffers from tubal disease or blockage, for instance due to endometriosis, but is also offered in cases where no apparent cause of infertility can be found – which seems astonishing. In few other branches of medicine is treatment offered which may be ineffective or simply fail because it is treating a symptom rather than the underlying cause. The high failure rates, linked to the high costs, should surely mean that IVF is only offered where the chances of success are high rather than as an action of first resort.

For many couples, IVF is the end of the road: if it doesn't work, they are likely to remain childless. The low success rates are startlingly grim. According to HFEA figures, in women aged less than 25, using their own eggs, the pregnancy rate per treatment cycle is 21.2 per cent, but with miscarriages taken into account this drops to 17.2 per cent. With improved career prospects and later marriage, many women do not discover their infertility until they are in their 30s. By the age of 35–9, the pregnancy rate drops to 16.7 per cent and the live birth rate to 13.1 per cent per cycle, and in the 40s the rate drops even more alarmingly. Older women are likely to have a higher success rate using donor eggs, but these are in short supply, and the use of donor eggs does not appeal to all women, some of whom prefer to try adoption or remain childless.

The process of IVF is stressful, both physically and emotionally. It involves the collection of eggs and sperm which are mixed outside the woman's body (hence the original popular term 'test-tube baby'). The resulting embryos are left to grow for a day or so, to check that they are developing normally, and then up to three (the legal maximum) are transferred into the woman's womb. If you produce many more embryos, then it may be possible to freeze some of them for later use if the first treatment fails, but frozen embryos do not always survive and there is a lower live birth rate. The procedure of egg collection is carried out under sedation or general anaesthetic.

As most women only release one egg per month, IVF is usually preceded by a course of drug treatment which causes the ovaries to mature several eggs in one monthly cycle; this is to increase the chance of producing several embryos. Some clinics prefer not to stimulate the ovaries in this way but collect the one egg produced naturally, because there are risks associated with stimulating ovulation, chiefly multiple pregnancy and ovarian hyperstimulation syndrome. This means that some women will develop a moderate over-response to the drugs and may develop cysts on the ovaries; the condition can be treated, after medical advice, with bed rest, good fluid intake and simple painkillers. The more severe form (which develops in about 1 per cent of cases) means that a very large number of eggs develop and the ovaries swell, causing alarming symptoms of nausea, vomiting, abdominal pain, shortness of breath, weakness, possible fainting and reduced urination – urgent hospital admission is then required.

As egg collection involves a minor operation, many IVF clinics prefer to collect more than one egg at a time. In this case drugs containing stimulating hormones are usually given. These will be in the form of a nasal spray or an injection (such as Buserelin); given every day throughout the 28-day cycle to suppress the natural levels of hormones produced during a normal menstrual cycle; an injection (HMG – human menopausal gonadatrophin, or FSH – follicle stimulating hormone) given once a day for the first half of the cycle, or tablets to stimulate ovulation; followed by ultrasound scanning which shows when an adequate number of eggs are maturing; and a final hormone injection (HCG –

human chorionic gonadatrophin) which completes the maturing process. This is timed 34 to 38 hours before egg collection, so that the eggs will be mature but will not have left the ovary. The injections will be given by the clinic or your GP, or may be self-administered – which cuts down on the inconvenience factor but involves training and the overcoming of squeamishness. Many women complain of experiencing the problems normally associated with menopause when taking these drugs: hot flushes, headaches, night restlessness, depression and irritability, which can make life extremely unpleasant.

Eggs are collected in one of two ways. Most commonly these days, ultrasound is used (under mild sedative), where a fine, hollow needle is passed through the bladder, urethra or vagina and each egg is removed in turn. It can be uncomfortable during and after the procedure and painkilling drugs may be needed. It is also common to lose a small amount of blood afterwards. Alternatively, a laparoscopy under general anaesthetic may be carried out (this has the increased risk of any procedure carried out under general anaesthetic). A small cut is made just below the navel for a laparoscope to be inserted and a fine hollow needle is again used to remove the eggs. Any associated pains and vaginal bleeding should disappear after a few days. The eggs are then mixed with the man's sperm in a dish in order to be fertilised.

ICSI (intracytoplasmic sperm injection) is a newer technique which has been developed and can help when the male partner has a low sperm count. It involves injecting a single sperm that has been identified as of sufficient quality into an egg retrieved from the woman, offering a greater chance of fertilisation. If it fertilises, the egg is transferred in the usual way, through the cervix into the womb using a catheter. If one or more of the embryos implants, then pregnancy develops. However, ICSI, introduced to Britain in 1993, has become increasingly controversial because genetic defects are more likely using this technique – fathers may effectively be passing their problem on to their sons (see p. 64).[9] However, this technique reduces the need to use sperm donors.

Very few people are totally sterile and most IVF cases will use the couple's own egg and sperm, but donated sperm is usually available. Donated eggs are a more difficult option because there are not very many women prepared to donate their eggs (egg donors are usually those who have completed their families), it is not a pain-free procedure and the eggs cannot be stored.

The future question?

Naomi Pfeffer raises various pertinent points about infertility and its treatment.[10] She argues that we have no way of knowing how widespread infertility is because not all couples seek medical help – they may choose not to investigate the problem; further, while they may regret the loss of their fertility in theory, they do not necessarily grieve the absence of a child. This is an interesting point when we discuss the 'right to a child' argument. Those who seek medical treatment are not necessarily those most desperate to have a child – they simply choose or are advised along the path of a medical solution to their problem. We may ask why parenthood is associated with the capacity to reproduce. Does everyone have a right to a child, when some people make appalling parents? Value judgements on this issue abound, but unfortunately our parenting skills are necessarily assessed in retrospect – it is almost impossible to forecast who will be an unsatisfactory parent.

The causes of infertility remain relatively unknown – in many cases couples find no medical reason why they should be infertile and IVF is generally offered as a possible solution in such cases. Despite technological changes, we seem no further on with discovering the true causes of infertility. If we can identify no cause for infertility for a number of couples, exactly why does IVF sometimes work? Generally, the problem is treated as physical even where there may be no physical cause. We know little of the socioeconomic make-up of infertile people, and whether social class, race, marital status come into the equation is impossible to define. We do know that there is differential access to health care generally, and there is no reason to believe that the working classes fare any better in fertility treatments than they do within the rest of health service provision, as highlighted in the now elderly Black Report (still pertinent, as the situation has not significantly changed since its publication in 1984).[11]

There is little agreement on the length of time it takes to become pregnant, but Pfeffer suggests that doctors involved in reproductive technology have a professional niche carved out for themselves – the work is exciting, high-status and technically complex; and it involves money. Although much of the treatment is unpleasant (for instance, the post-coital test) and often seemingly unscientific (such as performing IVF when the cause of infertility is unknown), such doctors are keen to treat according to their preference as a way of maintaining their position. Like most professionals, they wish to protect their own status, belief or stance by following a particular line of research or treatment to the exclusion of others. Therefore IVF may be offered where it is not necessarily the most appropriate form of treatment or without full prior investigation of the cause of infertility, a criticism made by some couples who have experienced the devastating feelings that failed IVF attempts can engender.

Very rarely are we fully critical of the infertility treatments available, and certainly most people who have undergone successful IVF will feel it is all worth it, but treatments have always been controversial. Drugs used to stimulate ovulation were introduced in the 1960s – even then there was concern about multiple births after the birth of sextuplets occurred. There were also questions concerning the safety of such medicines. In 1996 the Mandy Allwood case showed that little had really changed.[12] Many people who do not have to undergo infertility treatments are filled with revulsion by some of the techniques; so not only is infertility stigmatised, but its treatment as well. For example, AID (artificial insemination by donor) existed in the 1930s as a solution to male infertility but many people saw it as a veterinary technique which should be confined to farming. Today much of the controversy relates to the welfare of the embryos and concern about a market trade in human gametes.

Ethics

Janet Gallagher[13] tells us that in 1984 an American couple were killed in an air crash, leaving two frozen embryos immersed in liquid nitrogen in Australia. It raised a number of problems. Who owned them? Could they inherit? Did they have a right to life? Could they be donated, or thawed and allowed to die? Or should they be left in limbo? Who should make the decision? With the question marks about the destruction of frozen embryos in 1996 still resounding in our ears,[14] such extreme circumstances raise questions about the handling of human material outside the body and the types of parents now available – genetic, gestational and social. In early 1997 a woman, aged 52, gave birth by Caesarean section to her daughter's baby as a surrogate mother – her daughter was born without a womb. The genetic material was the daughter's and her husband's. The mother simply carried or incubated the baby and sustained a pregnancy for her daughter, and most people can see that mother love is the motive in this. All seems to have worked out well and people have been less damning of this case of surrogacy mainly because it involves a mother–daughter relationship rather than a financial deal between strangers, but what if there is a dispute? There have been a number of these in the USA and the outcome is generally a long court battle, with the welfare of the child seemingly forgotten despite the view that it should be paramount.

The superovulation necessary for IVF usually means some spare good eggs are left after the maximum of three are implanted. Usually, the spare embryos are frozen. After all the effort, simply to destroy them if they are not wanted later seems a poor option and, as we have mentioned, the issue created public uproar in 1996. Cryopreservation is fine if you perhaps want to try to bear another child later, but whose are these excess embryos? What if a couple divorces or has a dispute? The Warnock Commission in 1985 found the embryo had no legal status per se. In the USA an embryo is treated as a legal person, raising the spectre of future law suits. Cases seem to be growing increasingly extreme – American women have been jailed for adopting a lifestyle when pregnant which has contributed to the ill health of their babies. In America and the UK some women have been subjected to forced Caesareans despite their refusal to consent, because surgery has been deemed necessary for the health of the foetus. Where does the issue go from here? Could a child in later years sue its parents because of some alleged trauma sustained by being born after assisted conception techniques?

Michelle Stanworth raises the almost unthinkable issue of eugenics.[15] George Bernard Shaw, it is said, was excited by the prospect of using artificial insemination as a means of multiplying the offspring of a gifted minority. Most would-be parents do not think in such terms and generally have fine motives, but genetic knowledge has greatly accelerated and it is now possible to choose the qualities of our offspring to some extent, at least in terms of disability and also gender. Scientists have now identified over 3,000 conditions transmitted genetically from parent to offspring, from life-threatening diseases to minor afflictions. The basis is there (and to some extent is already used during unassisted pregnancy through techniques such as chorionic villi sampling (CVS) and amniocentesis) to make life or death choices during pregnancy on the basis of affliction. The Chinese one-child policy and cultural preference for high-status male children has meant that female foetuses are aborted; infanticide is practised in many rural areas of the country. The problem also exists in other parts of Asia, and even in Russia it appears to be considered acceptable to abort a foetus if it is the 'wrong' sex (which may mean male or female according to parental preference), a very worrying global misuse of ultrasonography techniques. Stanworth argues that there is a danger of the gene pool becoming more important than the welfare of the child. Within fertility treatments now there is potential for choosing which embryos are implanted and which rejected.

Has IVF subjected women to invasive and risky surgical procedures which might more properly be called experimentation? All procedures involving the use of general anaesthetic involve some risks, and most people would not opt for a general anaesthetic lightly. Arguably, with many patients not understanding the low success rates of IVF despite information offered by clinics and the counselling available, then it is still a form of experimentation.

Infertility becomes a feminist issue where women are seen in society in terms of their value as childbearers. Indeed, many of our contributors have expressed a feeling that they are not real women unless they can reproduce, so strong are the historical and cultural ties to childbearing as woman's main role. At a societal level, we need to examine why this is the case, why women are less valued for their many other capabilities, such as the ability to run a multinational company. As childbirth has become increasingly male-controlled, so has infertility treatment; and in this field too women are once again dominated by men.

Notes and references

1. Julia Stonehouse, *Idols to Incubators*, Scarlet Press, 1994.
2. Hilary Rose, 'The Politics of Reproductive Science', in Michelle Stanworth (ed.), *Reproductive Technologies: Gender, Motherhood and Medicine*, Polity Press, 1987.

3. Foresight was formed in 1978 to promote preconceptual care and to promote the study of aspects of the environment upon preconceptual health. Their preconception programme advocates following guidelines regarding diet; avoiding smoking, alcohol and street drugs; learning natural family planning methods; checking for (possibly hidden) genito-urinary infections and candida (thrush); providing help with allergies; and obtaining hair analyses to seek help with vitamin and mineral supplementation if indicated. The aim is that in future the NHS will help to take the programme forward as a major form of preventative care for couples wanting babies.

4. Stonehouse, *From Idols to Incubators*.

5. Theo Coburn, John Peterson Myers and Dianne Dumanoski, *Our Stolen Future*, Little, Brown, 1996.

6. Jacques Gélis, *History of Childbirth, Fertility, Pregnancy and Birth in Early Modern Europe*, trans. Rosemary Morris, Polity Press, 1991.

7. Ann Oakley, 'From Walking Wombs to Test Tube Babies', in Stanworth (ed.), *Reproductive Technologies*.

8. Juliette Zipper and Selma Sevenhuijsen, 'Surrogacy: Feminist Notions of Motherhood Reconsidered', in Stanworth (ed.), *Reproductive Technologies*.

9. A study into ICSI has been carried out by Dr Maryse Bonduelle at Brussels Free University, Belgium, and advocates counselling for parents undergoing this technique, although the risk of genetic defect remains low. In 1994, 253 British babies were born after the treatment, and it is estimated that 2,000 children in the UK today are the result of ICSI techniques. Professor Christine Gosden of Liverpool University has expressed concern about the infertile father passing on his own sperm problems and creating new mutations. The Medical Research Council's Genetics Unit in Edinburgh has shown that ICSI may be responsible for passing on genetic mutations of the male Y–chromosome which can cause infertility in boys.

10. Naomi Pfeffer, 'Artificial Insemination, In Vitro Fertilisation & the Stigma of Infertility' in Stanworth (ed.), *Reproductive Technologies*.

11. The Working Group on Inequalities in Health chaired by Sir Douglas Black, which produced the Black Report, basically looked at social inequalities in health – e.g. more

lower-working-class people smoke, they have poorer general health, the highest foetal and infant mortalities are associated with lower socioeconomic grouping. Evidence seems to show that little has changed since then; further research gathered during the 1990s shows that no significant policy changes have been made despite the evidence. ,

12. Mandy Allwood became pregnant as a result of fertility drugs given by her GP. Having not followed the GPs advice relating to abstention from intercourse during the drug treatment, she became pregnant with octuplets. The case was controversial for many reasons, not least because medical experts considered that she should selectively abort some of the embryos to give the others a chance of survival. This Ms Allwood refused to do and eventually all foetuses miscarried. There was also a cost element – all the babies, had they been born alive, would almost certainly have needed special care.

13. Janet Gallagher, 'Eggs, Embryos & Fetuses: Anxiety and the Law', in Stanworth (ed.), *Reproductive Technologies*.

14. Many embryos may be produced during IVF treatment, but clinics are allowed to replace only three, with many preferring to use only two. Most IVF clinics therefore have storage facilities so that spare embryos can be frozen for use in a later treatment cycle. This avoids the need for repeated drug stimulation, egg retrieval, sperm collection and fertilisation, and in some ways reduces the trauma of the treatment. The downside is that not all embryos survive freezing and the live birth rate from frozen embryos tends to be lower. If embryos are not needed they may be donated for the treatment of others or for use in research. They may also be allowed to perish. There was much controversy in the UK in 1996 when thousands of frozen embryos were destroyed – pro-life campaigners felt that the embryos should be treated as potential babies. A number of contributors to this book have questioned the degree of information they are given and the help they receive in making a decision regarding the freezing of embryos. It is an issue which needs careful consideration.

15. Michelle Stanworth, 'The Deconstruction of Motherhood', in Stanworth (ed.), *Reproductive Technologies*.

2 Infertility and its effects on relationships

Infertility and IVF treatment can lead to a number of relationship difficulties, both with a partner and with other people, such as friends. The following contributions eloquently express the difficulties which can arise when two partners react in different ways to a problem. COTS (Childlessness Overcome through Surrogacy) notes that 60 per cent of infertile couples eventually separate. Although many such relationships survive, it is easy to see how the cultural and societal expectations of fertility and personal recriminations and feelings that accompany its failure can wreck a relationship, especially where a couple undergo the trial of unsuccessful IVF treatments.

Rhonda
Our relationship has been very stressed. Every time we speak it is about IVF. I am ratty all the time. We argue. Sex goes out of the window. Everything we do is wrong, every time we talk about IVF we argue and tend to blame each other for having to go through the treatment. Gordon, my husband, could always just walk away and have a family with someone else, which worries me a lot as he's always wanted children.

Friends tend not to like telling you that they are pregnant – it does hurt, but you have to hide your feelings and tell them that you are pleased. I have a friend who can't have kids either. We would both love to see each other pregnant, but if only one of us did at least it would give the other some hope, but it would make me feel even more jealous and wonder why not me.

During a detailed interview, Cheryl, aged 31, and Andrew, aged 34, told very honestly of their experiences of three attempts at IVF (all of which failed) and the effects upon their relationship.

Cheryl and Andrew

We met in 1988 and married in 1989, then started trying for a baby immediately. After a year I was sent for tests. First was a laparoscopy, which discovered damaged tubes. I was given a dye test (a hysterosalpingogram), but no dye got through the tubes. I had tubal surgery to try to repair the damage, then tried to get pregnant. I requested another dye test before thinking about IVF; a little dye got through on one side.

Our first IVF attempt was done privately, which cost around £1,300. I didn't take in anything we were told at the time about failure rates, risks. In my mind, nothing was in proportion – I just couldn't have children.

When Cheryl started her hormone injections, the doctor thought she was slow to react and increased the dose. Cheryl panicked 'I thought I would have no children; I was going to die.'

Andrew, logically, highlighted five stages at which it is clear IVF has failed:

1. Failure to respond to the drugs.
2. Not producing (enough) eggs.
3. Eggs not fertilising.
4. Eggs not implanting.
5. Failed pregnancy test.

He was concerned that the statistics relating to IVF are not broken down enough. 'We felt that we were young, healthy and only suffered tubal problems, so we were more likely to be successful.'

Cheryl produced four eggs, two of which fertilised. They didn't 'take'. The couple left it for six months and then went privately once more for IVF. This time Cheryl produced eight eggs, but most didn't fertilise as they were not ripe enough. Andrew explained: 'There are only certain times and dates available for recovering eggs, so the eggs can be taken out at the wrong time – it is only known in retrospect.' The hospital they had chosen had no freezing facility. Three eggs were implanted. Cheryl explained her feelings at that time:

I felt more positive, but got so worked up and tunnel-visioned. Nothing else in life mattered. The world could have collapsed around me – I had lots of severe PMT, I was crying all the time and stressed out. I coped terribly and was offered counselling. Nothing happened and I had to return two weeks later to have the pregnancy test. We drove to the hospital in total silence. I had the test and was told to telephone for the result. I was told it was negative. It was horrid, not a nice way to tell anyone such news; I started my period and it floored me; it was awful.

The failed IVF hit Cheryl badly:

My GP was really good, but she has a little girl and she agreed she couldn't understand what it was like for me. I was offered tranquillisers. The two failed attempts so close together hit us badly. I hated everyone with children. The first attempt didn't bother me so much as I didn't get to the pregnancy test stage, but the second failure really hit me.

Andrew again mentioned the statistics and the role they have to play in people's expectations of the treatment:

What is needed is a very accurate assessment of the statistics. As we went along the process, we felt our odds increased as we hadn't fallen at the other hurdles. At implantation time we felt positive and thought we had a 50 per cent chance, so the sense of loss was much greater. We really need a national study offering information on the odds at each stage, whether they be one in ten or one in 250.

The couple couldn't face another IVF attempt immediately, so went on the NHS waiting list for their nearest hospital. After two years they were called in to an initial meeting with all the other couples in the area and attended a lecture by the consultant, who talked about the statistics and so on. This centre only implanted two eggs as policy, which made a 2–3 per cent difference in chances of success. Cheryl noted: 'They didn't mention the bad side, only the positive. One girl there was clueless – she thought IVF always succeeded.' Cheryl was told she needed to lose weight, from 11 stone (70 kilos) to 9st 6lb (60 kilos) for NHS IVF, and went to Weightwatchers. She got down to a size ten. She expected her third IVF attempt to fail, despite hoping otherwise. On this attempt Cheryl only produced six eggs but did have two embryos frozen. She was going to have her eggs put in some months later but kept putting it off, unable to face it:

I went for counselling as I was in tears all the time, very upset. I couldn't help feeling a failure, that there was something wrong; I wasn't normal. All my friends were able to have children, and people offered all sorts of folklore about relaxation. I tried it all.

When we went for counselling, we had already thought of adoption but didn't tell the hospital, scared they'd cancel the IVF. I met a woman at counselling. She was really nervous, her legs were shaking and she was chewing her fingers. She had had over 20 IVF attempts and refused to give up. I think she made me realise how bad it could get.

Cheryl tried alternative therapy, something called the Bowen technique, as she was frightened of failure through stress:

It was as if I had constant bad PMT – I was laid on a bed, face down in my undies. The woman touched me under my bra strap, on my neck and by my ears – I felt as if I was drunk, tingly and floaty. She did the same with my knees, tummy and neck and left me for ten minutes. Then I had to drink four glasses of water. I felt a different person, unbelievably relaxed. We went on holiday and we were accepted for adoption. I had reached 30 and my married life had been geared round an obsession; we needed quality of life. It affected our relationship and we needed to know whether we were having babies or not. For the last IVF, I felt more positive and as if it couldn't go on forever – I was sick of meeting women whose lives had been wrecked by this obsession to have a child. We need to have the strength to say that there is a world without children, and it is so hard to do.

Once again, Andrew was shocked by some logical inconsistencies:

Many couples try and re-try IVF until they are too old for adoption, or the chance of adoption. Childless couples want children, but adoption and IVF don't work together. For example, the person who counselled IVF patients didn't have access to information on adoption and we were never advised to consider it – her job was to get us through IVF.

Cheryl had felt adoption was another sign of failure, but

I got up one morning and thought, 'That's it.' I'd been obsessed; I'd fallen out with all my friends with children. One friend who was six months pregnant felt she couldn't tell me. It's pathetic really – I had been such a bitch that I had lost my friends. Adoption changed from being second best. I thought, 'If I can't have my own, let's have someone else's.' I began wondering whether to donate my frozen embryos, but it is not easy to forget the pain and put it all behind us.

While Cheryl felt she was in a black hole her husband was also feeling the strain: 'It affects the husband as much because you are living with the woman.' Andrew had children from his first marriage but didn't have access:

I got that thrown in my face all the time. Sometimes you feel as if you're only there to produce sperm. The sexual side became mechanical and tied to dates, but more than that: the baby became a spectre that Cheryl wanted. It didn't exist but became an entity – the concept became a reality and became encompassing. I was excluded. Instead of giving me affection, she was giving it to a baby that didn't exist. She put nothing into our relationship – she didn't talk to me. It was like living with someone handicapped – everyone always had to be understanding. In fact if Cheryl had been in a wheelchair I'd have felt the same, but at least people could have seen that. I hated what it did to us. In Cheryl's mind, a baby existed. It affected my happiness and our relationship broke down. We didn't communicate; she didn't know I was there. We weren't close and honest, and couldn't talk as she was always hysterical and in tears. We went through the motions of a relationship. In my mind, I had left her.

Cheryl freely admitted she wanted Andrew for his sperm: 'I wanted this baby.' Sexually, she didn't feel like a full woman.

I couldn't relax and enjoy making love; tension affected everything. I felt a failure. He bought me some nice underwear and I refused to wear it as I couldn't relate as a feminine woman. I was damaged goods, like having a mastectomy. Sex was one more demand. There was no point to sex when we couldn't have a baby.

Andrew added:

> You don't have a full-blown relationship. What's the point?
> Everything is on a backburner. It puts a stopper on your life and
> you don't allow yourself free time like holidays, Christmas. It
> was like carrying a sack of coal all the time. Everything we did
> had reduced satisfaction.

Andrew was a policeman whose work shifts added strain.

> We're easy going on the whole, but underneath there was a
> general unhappiness. I was unhappy because of how unhappy
> she was. No one dared speak about it. We could operate on a
> superficial level but we were unhappy with life and had an
> overwhelming sadness. We're so lucky to have been through
> it and to have come out OK.

Cheryl felt that if you are desperate, you will do anything for
a baby: 'I couldn't look at a pretty child – I couldn't relate to people
with children. Some friends came with their children, including
a beautiful little girl. I couldn't go near her – I couldn't touch or
go near her.' Andrew explained: 'This girl was the spectre
personified – the dream image come to life.'

Once the couple made a decision to leave the IVF treadmill and
aim for adoption, they were then caught up in the various
procedures involved in adoption vetting. They were ultimately
successful in being accepted for adoption, when Cheryl discovered
that she was pregnant naturally. Andrew in particular was highly
critical of the whole procedure:

> If a person is in constant pain, you have to accept this as a
> handicap or a medical problem. There is an underlying feeling
> from the medical profession that all is rosy. As soon as you are
> diagnosed as infertile, they offer treatment rather than treat the
> situation you are in. They don't examine the upset, depression,
> isolation, alienation and suffering that you experience from
> having no children – instead they try to give you children. It
> is not treated from the psychological side – the slant is wrong.
> The idea is: 'Infertile? Try IVF. Have faith – there's a baby out
> there, so go for it.'

The couple obviously had a very strong relationship; they had been to hell and back but survived it. Many do not. Interestingly, Cheryl is far from alone in becoming pregnant naturally after years of treatment for infertility and is critical that the causes of her problem were not examined thoroughly enough before IVF was recommended. Doctors interviewed confirmed that it is far from uncommon for patients finally accepted onto an IVF scheme after a long wait to withdraw having discovered their pregnancy – it is felt that the relief at being finally accepted for treatment allows the patient to relax, and nature takes its course. Much the same happens in instances like Cheryl's, where a patient finally accepts childlessness and starts to build a life without children.

Julie has had one successful IVF treatment where she carried triplets. One miscarried, but she gave birth to twin girls:

Julie
Before treatment I couldn't even bear to look at a baby and would actively avoid being in that situation. I also felt excluded as people would avoid discussing babies in front of me. Just knowing I'm infertile is very frustrating, as I am now with a new partner and feel inadequate in that I can't give him a baby of our own in the conventional way. With my previous partner, sex was the main thing affected. It was no longer an enjoyable experience; it was purely a method of getting pregnant. It became a mechanical act and I couldn't go back to enjoying it. I eventually only saw him as a necessary object to help me have a baby. This obviously was a problem for my husband and was subsequently a factor in our eventual break-up. With my present partner, sex is free of any underlying expectations and therefore completely enjoyable. I would be happy to have this treatment again to have another baby with my new partner but am scared of having another multiple pregnancy. While I wouldn't be without my twin daughters, I couldn't cope with twins or more again. If I was guaranteed to have only one child per pregnancy, then I would probably do it again.

Michelle and Graham's experience of IVF was extremely disappointing. Michelle has blocked and blown (severely scarred) tubes and a misshapen womb.

Michelle

The treatment brought us much closer together afterwards – you get through IVF, you can get through anything. It put so much pressure on, though – we had rows over silly things. I blocked Graham out because I was having the treatment. He only had a little (but important) bit to do. I felt I'd let him down when we found out it was my problem that stopped us having babies and told him he didn't have to stay. I'm now waiting for tubal surgery, but it's a year's wait so we're both hoping this will work.

Graham added: 'The pressure on the male is tremendous, mainly because you have so little actual involvement. Being supportive all the time brings its own problems. I sometimes felt I didn't exist because the treatment overtook our lives completely.'

Keith was born without the tubes leading from the testicles to the penis, so he cannot pass sperm during ejaculation. His wife, Lesley, was six months pregnant as the result of an IVF attempt at the time of writing. She explained how IVF affected their sex life:

Lesley

I did go off sex. This was mainly to do with the fact that when you go for monitoring you have to have an internal scan, so that they can check on the size and amount of eggs that are growing. I felt I had been messed about enough down there and didn't feel I could let Keith get close to that part. This was hard for Keith to understand, so left him feeling unloved, unwanted and very frustrated. After the treatment it was as if a great weight had been lifted.

Kathleen has occluded (blocked) fallopian tubes. She is currently undergoing her third IVF cycle.

Kathleen

It would be impossible to explain exactly how empty, useless, depressing and frustrating it is to have the potential parts of a female and not be able to have a much yearned for and longed for child. I have suffered for eleven years, one month at a time. Although my husband has been as desperate as me, if not more desperate, there have been times during the treatments when I have been intolerable as I was so wound up (it's like PMT but 20 times worse). The anxiety and frustration, along with the disappointments, put a great strain on us on several occasions.

Lorraine and John, who have already suffered one ectopic pregnancy, explained their desire for a baby and their relationship:

Lorraine
My personal desire for a baby is very hard to explain. It's something that I want so badly that I can't believe I'm ever going to get it. I can't imagine life without ever having a baby, and to see pregnant women and newborn babies all the time makes it even harder. When I see babies on TV or in the street, I get a deep feeling in my stomach which just tears me apart and I do my utmost not to cry. When you've been trying for a baby for five years you would think it would get easier, but I still feel the same every month when I get my period. I'm still hopeful that I'll get pregnant naturally, even though I know that we need IVF, but I can't give up hoping because that's the only thing that keeps me going. I want to be pregnant, I want to know how it feels to be kicked by an unborn baby, I want to give birth, to hear it cry. Just to hold and touch my own baby would be out of this world.

John is one of five children, who all have children except for him and Lorraine. 'We really would love a baby of our own, to be called Mum and Dad instead of Auntie and Uncle.'
The couple have a strong relationship:

John
I love Lorraine just as much as when we were first married, but after she lost the baby she needed loads of tender loving care. I couldn't cope with some of the things Lorraine had to do to herself (e.g. needles). I thought she was so brave.

John's mother had died two weeks before Lorraine's frightening ectopic pregnancy, which left him with a compounded sense of loss.
One contributor, awaiting IVF, explained how her relationships had been affected:

Anon

The whole issue of infertility is an emotional minefield. Because I haven't told many people, friends and relatives often say things which hurt. Some ask direct questions about when we're going to have a baby; others make tactless remarks about how fertile they are. I found the secrecy too much to handle and told my Mum. She was great (apart from telling me to relax and it would happen). Although it hasn't placed too much of a strain on the marriage, the weight of my problem is also borne by John and I felt I had to tell someone not directly involved to share the burden. Although my husband is very supportive, it is our problem, not just mine, and I was leaning on him too much and not appreciating how disappointed he is.

I have been through phases of outrage at people's questions and comments. His sister is particularly hard to handle. She keeps asking when we'll have a baby. I am now avoiding John's family, but I don't want to feel forced to divulge something that is private. I know I'm not relaxed and that may be playing a part in my failure to conceive. I have tried deep relaxation and am going to try reflexology. I'm too aware of things, but I cannot get having a baby out of my mind. I am used to controlling my life. Oddly enough, seeing babies didn't bother me for ages because I wanted my own conception and pregnancy. Now I look at babies and think, 'I want one.' Because the IVF treatment is two to three years away, I'm trying to come to terms with being childless. That may be the wrong thing to do, and maybe I should be hopeful for the future treatment, but I have to survive in the meantime.

I still haven't decided whether to tell people or not. They can be so tactless even when meaning well. It's funny how the issues of freedom not to have children, privacy and fulfilment in life weren't issues until we couldn't conceive.

Infertility affects people, and especially women, regardless of their other achievements in life. A woman can be academically successful and develop a good career, but will still feel the weight of being unable to bear children very heavily:

Anon

I am a social worker by profession and therefore trained to assist and counsel other people with their problems. Somehow because of this, I feel I ought to be able to cope with my own problems. For the most part, with the help of a very supportive husband, I have coped reasonably well with the trials and tribulations of the last six years. The yearning for a child is one that will never diminish completely, although as each year passes the reality of it ever happening becomes beyond reach.

I was diagnosed as having endometriosis and had surgery to remove large cysts and part of each ovary. This was followed by a course of Synorel and a battle to pursue IVF – to obtain funding on the NHS. Our first IVF treatment was undergone. I tried not to become too hopeful, because of the low success rate, but once the three embryos were implanted it was difficult not to believe they were babies. Sadly, not only was the IVF unsuccessful, but because of an infection contracted during one of the delicate procedures I became seriously ill with septicaemia [blood poisoning] and was admitted to hospital two months later.

As a result, I am naturally very apprehensive about further IVF. However, I do have frozen embryos remaining at the clinic and hope that one day I will feel able to pursue treatment.

The professionals at the clinic broke the news to us that the pregnancy test was negative in a very sensitive way – answering any questions we had and leaving us alone together for a while. As we walked out of the interview room after being informed of the results, there was a couple with a young baby – obviously one of the clinic's successes, but it seemed to make our failure seem much worse.

I feel that professionals jump to conclusions about couples' feelings and emotions following IVF treatment. When attending my local hospital for investigations for my illness following IVF, I was seen by a doctor who, prior to any tests, declared that in his opinion my physical symptoms were due to my emotional reaction to the failure of the IVF and that I needed to see a psychiatrist. I was appalled because I knew there was something seriously wrong with me physically. I had a raging temperature, had lost 1½ stone [9.5 kilos] in weight, had blackouts, etc. – this was the septicaemia. It took several months for me to recover, and today my partner and I tend to take life as it comes.

For any couple unable to conceive, a number of issues are raised within the text of this book, mainly emanating from couples who have been through the treadmill of treatments. Many are hopeful, and the first message is that couples shouldn't give up hope, even when the odds are stacked against them, but perhaps the overriding message is that in order to cope with the inevitable strains – physical, emotional, psychological – of infertility and its treatment, many couples need to know about the techniques, the issues, the experiences of others in order to make informed decisions at the outset of treatment. It can be very hard to come off the treadmill of treatments when hope is ever-present, but easier perhaps to make a decision at the start about how much invasive technology you wish to submit to in an attempt to have a child. Perhaps if all parents had to think so hard about the subject of parenting, then the position of both women and children worldwide would be improved.

Shari Thurer makes the comment that 'one of the great puzzles of our history is that ... a blatant disregard of women and children coincided with the greatest glorification of mother and child.'[1]

Note

1. Shari L. Thurer, *The Myths of Motherhood: How Culture Reinvents the Good Mother*, Penguin, 1995.

3 Medical issues behind infertility

The chances of pregnancy

The World Health Organisation defines infertility as the failure to conceive after one year of unprotected intercourse, but only around 85 per cent of couples will conceive within this time. The figure rises to 90 per cent after two years. So, the chance of conception is thought to be 25 to 30 per cent per menstrual cycle. There are then 10 per cent of couples who are unlikely to achieve conception within the two-year time period, and even after intensive investigation no specific cause will be found to explain the infertility of 10–20 per cent of these couples.

Where causes are diagnosed, the most common fertility issues are problems with ovulation, or tubal damage in women and sperm dysfunction in men.

For anyone planning a baby, preconceptual care is of supreme importance. Many women now know that daily folic acid supplements are recommended to lower the risk of their baby developing spina bifida, but couples should also stop smoking (or reduce as far as possible) and limit alcohol intake, as both tobacco and alcohol may affect the ability to conceive to some degree. Women who are very heavy or too light may experience menstrual irregularities and are often advised to try to attain a certain weight level. Some couples will have already been trying to direct lovemaking towards ovulation time, but ovulation can be difficult to predict and making love regularly is more likely to be successful. Ovulation prediction kits are available (at a cost), and some women are now using the Persona contraceptive kit (available from leading chemists) to highlight the times when they are likely to be fertile – the effectiveness of such measures is not yet known. Moreover, Foresight will analyse a hair sample from a prospective parent and provide an analysis of any deficient or superfluous minerals and vitamins which may be relevant in dealing with subfertility.

There are fairly straightforward tests which may be carried out in the early stages of consultation. For men, a sperm analysis may be used; for women, a blood test on day 21 of the menstrual cycle can check progesterone level and whether ovulation has occurred. If these tests are satisfactory, then the fallopian tubes may be tested. This is done by hysterosalpingogram (an X-ray visualisation of dye passing through the tubes), or more recently by Echovist (an equivalent technique which uses ultrasound), or by the more invasive laparoscopy and dye checks. For the first two procedures it is possible to be treated as an out-patient; the other involves admission to hospital and anaesthetic.

To stimulate ovulation if necessary, a drug called Clomiphene is often used in amounts ranging from 50 mg to 150 mg. This will start many women ovulating but ironically, may prevent conception by thickening the cervical mucus, so that it acts as a barrier to sperm. Other agents can be tried (by injection), such as gonadatrophin hormones which require careful measurement because of fears of hyperstimulation of the ovaries. These drugs have side effects and risks which should be fully discussed with medical staff.

Male infertility can be harder to deal with and usually IVF, sub-zonal insemination (SUZI – where a single sperm is injected into the egg itself) or ICSI is suggested. In some cases, where there are problems with the sperm, donor insemination may be an answer, or possibly adoption if donor sperm does not appeal.

Pelvic inflammatory diseases (PID)

Today over 40 per cent of the incidences of infertility in women can be put down to blocked tubes and pelvic adhesions. Endometriosis, covered in detail later in this chapter, is itself a major cause of tubal problems.

Pelvic infections which lead to a fertility problem have three main causes: sexually transmitted diseases; a disease acquired at the time of abortion, miscarriage or delivery; or peritonitis, most commonly due to appendicitis. It is important that women should understand that tubal blockages discovered during medical checks are not necessarily a hangover from venereal disease, with all the associated stigma.

Sexually transmitted diseases

A good deal of fallopian tube blockage is caused by pelvic infection, commonly chlamydia (an extremely aggressive bacterial organism which directly invades the pelvic cavity). Often women do not know they have any such infection and there are frequently no symptoms, as contributors to this book will testify. Rather than subjecting women to invasive operations on their fallopian tubes which may be unsuccessful or, if successful, lead to a greater risk of ectopic pregnancy, the answer may lie in education. For young women embarking on their early sexual experiences, it would be worth extolling the virtues of barrier contraception, since chlamydia, like almost all pelvic inflammatory diseases, is venereal, meaning sexually transmitted. Where pelvic infection is discovered, prompt treatment may help to avoid problems later. The few symptoms which may be noticeable are reddening and soreness of the vagina and perhaps a burning sensation on urination. Chlamydia is possibly the most dangerous of all the organisms that can invade the female pelvic cavity. It insidiously destroys the lining of the fallopian tubes and creates extensive scar tissue throughout the pelvic cavity. This can ruin a woman's reproductive organs without her ever knowing she has the infection.

Other infections

Not all pelvic infections are venereal; there can also be an invasion from inside the pelvic cavity. A bout of appendicitis in childhood may itself be responsible for severe scarring in the tubes and other reproductive organs, and peritonitis, which is a rare complication of appendicitis, can leave behind an infection that causes tubal blockage. It is also well documented that pregnant women can develop a similar infection at the cessation of their pregnancy.

Lyn

During my first marriage I gave birth, naturally, to two wonderful children. Soon after my second marriage, however, I learned that a pelvic infection years earlier had blocked my fallopian tubes beyond repair, making another pregnancy impossible. At first we could not believe that we would not have a baby together, even though we were lucky enough to have and love my two children, whom my husband later went on to adopt. At this stage I was still only 26 years old and had always wanted a big family.

It was only when my GP suggested IVF that we finally saw a ray of hope, although we were disappointed to learn that it would be about 18 months before we could see a consultant, and then up to another two years before the actual treatment could begin. We tried to get on with our lives, but I couldn't help but feel pangs every time a friend or neighbour became pregnant.

When our first IVF attempt came we were both excited and worried. The treatment itself was very stressful – so much to remember, different drugs to take and so many emotions and expectations. I found the daily injections very painful and my arms ached from all the blood tests, but I kept thinking that it would all be worthwhile. The day of egg collection arrived and we were very excited. They collected eight eggs and we went home elated – I slept better than I had in a long time. Next day we were told that two eggs were very good and would be replanted. This was very simple and not at all painful, and when they gave us a scan of our two embryos we both cried. When my period arrived nine days later, our dream was shattered. We all cried, including our two children. We had tried to keep the stress away from them, and to prepare them for disappointment, but they were just as upset as we were.

I felt a complete failure – my husband was wonderful, telling me how brave I had been to undergo all that treatment and that I should be proud of myself, but it was a long, long time before I could feel anything like pride.

Our second attempt followed the same pattern as the first, two years later. Once again we were full of hopes, and again we were bitterly disappointed when it failed, and a little angry this time too, that we could give a baby so much love and time, and a wonderful family, and again it wasn't to be. Again we tried to get on with our lives and we threw ourselves into our family and into voluntary work. The pain was always there, though, and the desperate longing for a baby.

By the time of our third attempt we had been trying for nearly ten years. Some of our friends and family were concerned that we were putting ourselves through it all again and wondered how we would cope if it failed, but we had no qualms – my husband said that when I had had enough we would know to stop.

The third attempt failed too, although the treatment had all the potential for success – it just wasn't to be. Once again we were left empty and baby-less, and nothing could console us or ease the deep pain we felt.

Now, three months on, the pain is still there, as is the desire, but once again we have to pick up the pieces for our two children's sake. Life is precious and for living. We are waiting to see if we can have another attempt – we won't give up till the very last.

Derek Tuffnell, consultant obstetrician and gynaecologist at Bradford Royal Infirmary, sees IVF not just as a treatment, but as a diagnostic tool in its own right – if a couple, with help, can produce a good egg and a good sperm, but the two fail to form an embryo, then that in itself is a valid indicator that, genetically, these two people should perhaps be advised against further attempts at reproduction. He always suggests a maximum of three attempts at fertilisation. If fertilisation is successful, but the embryo fails to implant, then he suggests an absolute maximum of two further attempts, beyond which he firmly believes in listening to the body and following other avenues.

Rhonda suffered tubal damage due to PID and did consider adoption.

Rhonda
We're in a Catch 22 situation because we live in a one-bedroom house; the council won't move us until we have children; the adoption people won't let us adopt because we haven't got room.

Instead, Rhonda and husband Gordon have tried IVF and are awaiting their second treatment. Rhonda explained her feelings during treatment:

Before, we felt very apprehensive, excited and worried. During, I felt very tired, irritable, moody, tearful; sometimes I felt like I wanted to stop the treatment, that I didn't have a life outside hospital. After, my emotions were mixed – we were relieved that the treatment was finished, but disappointed that it hadn't worked: I felt empty. The only really good reason we would give up treatment would be if it endangered my life, but, going through a cycle, I can see how easy it would be to stop through stress.

Helen, our next contributor, put the case for never giving up hope.

Helen
Eight years ago I suffered an ectopic pregnancy and was told that the chances of my becoming pregnant again were slim. Several years of trying finally led us to a fertility clinic where I was diagnosed as having suffered from a pelvic infection, leaving me with only fragments of fallopian tube. We were absolutely devastated, and understood that IVF was our only remaining hope.

Helen and her husband went on to have two unsuccessful IVF attempts, followed by two further attempts where the eggs failed to fertilise:

My family and friends were involved at all times and were very supportive – without them the years of agony would have been unbearable. Throughout all this, your life is upside down – you live, eat and breathe IVF, and your relationship with your husband must be very strong because it pushes you to your limits, emotionally, financially and physically.

At this stage the fertility clinic regretfully stated that they could do nothing further to help, and suggested that perhaps there was a problem with Helen's eggs: 'Talk about feeling like a failure.' But Helen refused to give up:

We sought help financially, as we had used up all of our savings. I also took up yoga and meditation, had counselling which I needed very badly, and changed my diet to a more healthy one, giving up all alcohol. At least then I could tell myself that there was nothing more I could do.
    For our fifth attempt (at a different clinic) I was put on twelve ampoules of Perganol to increase the number of follicles.

The egg collection produced eight eggs, four of them Grade A, all of which fertilised, and three were implanted. The next two weeks were hell, but for us it was fifth time lucky – the pregnancy test was positive, and later a scan showed two heartbeats. I can't tell you the joy we felt. Peter and Matthew were born, fit and well, nine months later.

I want to tell others never to give up hope – fight on and you just might get there. Counselling really helped me, and I can't recommend it highly enough.

The media make IVF out to be so easy – but it's not, it's very hard, and my heart goes out to people who still have to go through it. There can be such a huge gap in your life that nothing other than a baby can fill, and nobody knows the heartache you go through, because it's too painful to describe.

Mandy wrote to us with a lengthy diary which we wish we had space to print in full. The following are key extracts from her story so far.

Mandy

When you've been trying for a child for over three years, had endless blood and sperm tests and spent six months on fertility drugs, with no result, you know something is seriously wrong. I think in a way I'll be glad if they find some reason for our inability to conceive; at least then we'll know what we have to deal with.

We learn that the laparoscopy has shown that both my fallopian tubes are badly blocked. Having read enough books I know exactly what that means. 'Can you do anything?' is all I can say. No, the extent of blockage is too great and the success rate for an operation to try to clear them is only around 2 per cent.

We discuss the options open to me and IVF is recommended as my only real hope of having a baby. I think deep down I expected this.

Stupid thoughts go through my head. I even tell Carl to divorce me so he can find a 'real woman'. His reaction surprises me: he tells me he loves me and married me for that reason. With or without kids, we will always be together. We talk about IVF and both agree that no matter what the cost we will try anything.

We're lucky that with the medical steps that have been made we can be helped. I know the success rate isn't brilliant, but after talking we have agreed to give IVF a try. It isn't a magic cure, but we know we have to try, no matter what.

Three weeks later we also enquire about adoption; we feel it's best to explore all the avenues open. Neither of us can imagine a life without children and should the IVF fail then adoption will be the only other option open to us.

We are visited a couple of weeks later by a representative from the adoption agency. They are unable to consider us as prospective adoptive parents for a child over twelve months old until we have gone down the IVF road. Should that be unsuccessful we will be eligible for consideration. We can, however, go on the waiting list for a baby. Because of the shortage of babies being put up for adoption and the length of the waiting list we can apply, as it would probably take at least a couple of years before they could take our initial application any further, by which time we may already have tried and failed with IVF and would then be eligible for consideration.

We have a brief discussion and the doctor confirms that both my fallopian tubes are blocked. All I want to know is what has caused this, and the only explanation is that I must have had an infection sometime in the past without knowing about it.

Considering I have always been scrupulous about having regular smear tests, I want to know why nothing has ever been picked up on. I don't recall ever having any symptoms of something being wrong, apart from a time some seven years ago when I continually suffered from abdominal pain for a period of around three months. I consulted my family doctor at the time and despite swab tests and other investigations nothing was found. I was finally sent for an ultrasound, but again the results came back negative and my problem was then diagnosed as colic. Dr Palmer states that sometimes an infection can occur so high up that a normal swab or smear test would not pick it up.

Dr Palmer explains that there is no waiting list for IVF treatment in our area; perhaps this is because the treatment is not funded by our health authority and only those with the means to pay for treatment are in fact getting any help.

Attended meeting at the clinic. It was quite a surprise to see so many couples there. Infertility still seems to be a taboo problem and I guess Carl and I have felt very isolated since my diagnosis. The meeting consisted of a slide show and talk on the process of IVF, after which questions were raised and answers given. Neither of us really had any idea that the process was so complicated, not to mention expensive.

We have been told that it may be possible to have the required drugs prescribed by our family doctor, so saving £350. Not all fundholding GPs are prepared to offer this assistance – ours said yes. He will back us as much as possible. He even gave me the impression that he will support any necessary future attempts, which is fantastic.

So, Mandy and Carl are moving forwards into the unknown world of IVF and all that it brings with it.

Ovulatory failures

At least 50 per cent of the fertility problems in women are related to the production and release of eggs. The egg may not mature properly, or may not be correctly released. Ovarian release is controlled by the hormonal system, which may undergo disturbance.

The most common cause of serious ovulatory disorders is polycystic ovarian disease (PCO), where the ovaries become clogged with cysts and as a result rarely, if ever, release eggs. In many cases, women with PCO respond well to a course of superfertility drugs. Clomiphene citrate (Clomid), introduced in the early 1960s, can induce ovulation in nearly 80 per cent of all women with ovulatory failure.

Margaret
My story started some 16 years ago, when I got engaged. I saw a gynaecologist as my periods had always been rather scanty and irregular. As I was only 19, his reply was, 'You're too young to be worrying – you have to be 40 before you start worrying about starting a family.'

After our marriage we just hoped that nature would take its course. My periods continued to be completely irregular: sometimes very light, at other times very heavy, lasting for weeks or even months, and once with two years between periods. At last I was referred to a lady gynaecologist at the local hospital, who carried out various tests. Nothing was discovered. Finally I was referred to a leading hospital where I was told that I had polycystic ovaries – something which nobody had ever mentioned to me before. We were told of various treatments, more tests were carried out, and we were asked to return three months later. On our next visit there were yet more tests, and then we were told that we would be put forward for ovulation induction, a type of mini-IVF.

I was told to call the hospital on the first day of my next period, which I did. On the second day I had a scan, and then started on a series of daily injections which my husband could give. Over the next couple of weeks, regular visits were made to monitor the development of the ovaries. Nothing seemed to happen, so after three weeks it was decided to abandon the attempt and begin again on the next cycle with a higher dose.

The next time I hyperstimulated, and so the project was abandoned again. It was decided at this point to use drugs to switch off my own cycle – this was maintained for seven cycles. Sometimes nothing happened, but mostly I hyperstimulated.

Finally in March 1995 one doctor said 'You need IVF; then all follicles can be emptied and the eggs collected.' This was discussed with my husband, who (like me) wasn't too sure, but we knew it was our only chance. He had to give a sperm sample to check his suitability, which thankfully was fine. We applied to the local health authority for funding, which they agreed to give for two attempts.

My first cycle started in October 1995, taking a 'sniffer' [nasal spray] three times a day at 7am, 3pm and 11pm. After three weeks I went back for a scan and a blood test to check the hormone levels were low. The following day I started three injections of Perganol a day. Visits were made to the hospital every couple of days to check the stimulation and on day eleven it was decided my egg collection would be on day 13. My last 'sniff' was to be on day eleven at 11pm, along with another injection called Profasi, timed to be 36 hours before my egg collection. This was to be at 20 past midnight. This was to prime the eggs for collection. Finally on 7 November I had my egg collection, resulting in 27 eggs as my ovaries had hyper-stimulated. After a short time we left, leaving my eggs to be mixed with my husband's sample which had been given that morning. Because of the number of eggs my ovaries had swelled so much, causing a lot of pain and discomfort. On 9 November we returned to be told that only two eggs had fertilised and although I was still in some discomfort we were advised to have both implanted. They had been graded as Grade 1 and Grade 2.

We then had two weeks to wait for the result, just using Cyclogest pessaries for the next 15 days. This is the hardest time, as you feel in limbo. At last a blood test was taken, which gave a positive result but the hormone level was low. Two days later this was repeated to show that the level had trebled. I was pregnant. However, the joy was shortlived as a week later I started to show a brown discharge. Hormone levels were checked and still found to be going up, but only slowly. All we could do was to wait. After nine days of the discharge I started to bleed heavily and finally the following day I miscarried. I was devastated, to say the least. All my dreams seemed to have ended. Christmas 1995 was nothing like I had thought it would be a couple of weeks earlier. I thought I could never go through that again.

In January 1996 we returned to see the doctor to discuss the future. I told her I felt I couldn't go through it again, but what she said was the most important thing to me: 'You can get pregnant. We just need to maintain it.' I felt very mixed up, but when she told us she would be more hopeful next time we decided to have another try – there was still some funding. It was planned for February.

Again we started the sniffing and injections. This time it was Metrodin. After two and a half weeks nothing seemed to be happening, and at three weeks the cycle was abandoned to start again two weeks later. I asked to go back on Perganol. It worked! I had my last sniff at 11pm and my Profasi at 11.40pm. On Easter Saturday my egg collection resulted in 23 eggs, but without the pain and discomfort this time. I dreaded going back on Easter Monday in case nothing had fertilised but thankfully six had. It was decided that three would be transferred. Two Grade 1s and one Grade 2. Again we had a two-week wait. I was very nervous at the blood test as I dreaded the result. However, at 3.30pm, the allotted time, I rang. Positive again and with a high hormone level. All I could do was ask the sister to check the results again and again to make sure they were my results. Two days later another blood test confirmed that the levels were still rising. At 28 days after egg collection a scan confirmed one egg sac. We could hardly believe it. At 42 days a scan showed a foetus with a healthy beating heart. It was so clear that we could only stare in wonder. As they were happy with the results, they discharged me back to my own GP for antenatal appointments and a baby due on 28 December.

I have since had two more scans but still find it so hard to believe, even though the heartbeat can now be heard and my clothes are getting tight. I cannot possibly put into words the gratitude I feel for the IVF unit. They have given us the greatest Christmas present we could ever have wished for.

Linda's problem was not ovulating. She has had two gamete intrafallopian transfer (GIFT) treatments, six unsuccessful treatments and one successful IVF treatment, with the result that she has twin girls. These were all NHS treatments. She explained her desire for a baby with real feeling:

Linda
It was both a physical and emotional yearning. I wanted 'our' child. Adoption was put on our list of options by my doctor, but it was never on my list. Thankfully, I will never know if I'd go down that road. Emotions have a habit of taking over and, in the end, I imagine you'll do anything.

My infertility made me do things I would never have dreamed of: three 'A' levels and three years of a part-time degree. All my efforts went into my work. I had seven years of treatment in all and will never forget how it felt to be childless. Weddings, christenings (particularly) and Christmas all took their toll on our smiling mask. The arrival of my mother's first grandchild by my younger sister is a bleak time I will never forget. When my best friend married ten years after me and conceived almost straight away, I began to wonder what we had done to deserve such treatment.

Stigma is still attached to infertility. We helped organise a dance to support the Fertility Fund – we could not sell the tickets – all those infertile people in one place, a real no no. It was almost like coming out.

Early diagnosis of Stephanie's illness could have prevented months of fruitless attempts at conception, with its accompanying frustration.

Stephanie
Three years ago I discovered a small painful lump on the left side of my stomach. This was later diagnosed as a swollen

ovary caused by a cyst. I was told that nothing could be done and that the problem would go away. Each month around ovulation time the lump and the pain recurred and each month I suffered horrendously painful periods. This went on for approximately 18 months and, having taken no contraception since Roger and I married five years before, I began to suspect that something was not quite right. In June of last year we attended the gynaecology department of the local women's hospital. Here we underwent various tests and it was decided that I should start taking the fertility drug Clomid to boost ovulation. Three more months passed and still no results. Finally, a test in January of this year showed a blockage and a distortion in my left fallopian tube and a possible blockage in my right. It was after this discovery that we were referred to the fertility clinic.

In February of this year we had an initial meeting with one of the doctors. It was decided that we would pay for one cycle and if that was not successful the NHS would fund the cost.

Roger and I are a very private couple and made the decision to go through IVF without confiding in family or friends. At this stage we believed it to be a very straightforward procedure and we adopted a very matter-of-fact attitude towards it.

In April of this year the IVF treatment was started. I was on the long protocol treatment which involved up to four weeks of injections, blood tests and scans. It was at this stage that I began to experience the stress of IVF. The main problem was trying to juggle my job with the treatment, trying to sneak off for blood tests and scans without any of my colleagues finding out what was going on. The week prior to egg collection I visited my GP. He believed that the stress I was under could result in the treatment not working. I was not in a position to take any holiday leave, so he suggested that I should be signed off with an illness until the treatment was complete.

Egg collection took place on Saturday 11 May. To everyone's delight, twelve eggs were collected and Roger and I were sent home with instructions to return on the Monday for embryo replacement.

The following Monday we were given the horrifying news that none of the collected eggs had successfully fertilised. The doctor was very kind and sympathetic. However, his words did not mean a lot to me as this new world of fear engulfed me – the thoughts of being childless for ever kept going round and round in my head.

The next day Roger and I returned to the clinic for another meeting with the doctor. This time I listened carefully to what he had to say. We were told that we could pay for another treatment and still be entitled to NHS funding if that one did not work. The next treatment would be different and would involve a technique called ICSI where the sperm is injected directly into the egg to assist fertilisation. We were told to go away and think about what we wanted to do and to return for a follow-up appointment once I had had my next period. Following this meeting, doubts were sown into our minds. Why wasn't the ICSI technique used in the first instance? Why were we now allowed to pay for two cycles and still be eligible for NHS funding? We did not feel very positive about going through another treatment. However, we could see no alternatives.

No one could have prepared either of us for the onslaught of emotions which we experienced over the next few weeks. I found myself crying every time I was alone. I began to feel as though someone close to me had died, then I felt guilty because if someone had died it would be much worse. I was very confused and often found myself getting angry at Roger and blaming him for our predicament. We finally decided to confide in our families and a couple of close friends. It really was too heavy to handle this on our own. However, I still found it difficult to talk to outsiders. I did not understand my own emotions and could not expect others to understand what we were going through. Looking back, I was in desperate need of some counselling. I needed to talk to someone who understood. We were not offered any by the clinic and we both felt very alone in dealing with the emotional side of failure.

During my treatment I was following the TV series *Making Babies*. This I found fascinating and very informative. Sadly, after the treatment failed I found it quite unbearable to watch. However, I did read the book *Making Babies* written by Professor Winston and found this helped me to understand the emotions I was experiencing. Having read the book, everything seemed to be so much clearer. I now understood a lot more about IVF and realised how little I knew when we first set out. I felt it had given me some additional strength to see us through another

IVF attempt. I sent Professor Winston a short letter, thanking him for writing such a sympathetic and sensitive account of IVF.

When my period arrived, I felt that the sun had just come out. I realised that I had been suffering from severe PMT. This had made everything seem so black and so depressing. This, I discovered afterwards, is a side effect of the drugs I had been taking. I called the clinic to arrange our follow-up appointment.

It was decided that my next treatment should take place in July. I was a little worried that this was too soon, both physically and emotionally. However, we were so desperate to find out if we could get over the fertilisation problem that I agreed to it. Both Roger and I were united in our fear that the eggs would not fertilise. In fact, Roger was quite convinced they would not. We spent a great deal of time discussing this and being very open with each other. It really brought us very close together.

Egg collection took place on Friday 26 July. Eight eggs were collected. We had to wait until 12.30 the following day to establish if they had been fertilised. Saturday morning seemed to take forever to pass. It was one of the worst mornings of my life. When I called the clinic, they gave me the good news. Five eggs fertilised. Roger and I were so relieved. I really cannot put into words how we felt on receiving that news.

On the following Monday, two embryos were replaced and the remaining three embryos were frozen. By the Thursday I began to suspect that my period was on its way. I was suffering from the same PMT as before. By the following Thursday I was disappointed to discover that my period had actually arrived. The next day (14 days after egg collection) my pregnancy test results came back as expected – negative. I was surprised at how well both Roger and I handled the news. However, as we were expecting the worst the results we received compared quite favourably.

We looked upon this time as our first IVF attempt, and having studied the available statistics we accept that the chances of a first-time success are quite slim. Therefore we feel quite positive and have the confidence to try again.
Watch this space!

Our next contributor, diagnosed early as suffering from polycystic ovaries, was finally found to have even more complications.

J.A.

We decided to try for a family straight after our marriage, particularly since I had been diagnosed as having polycystic ovaries when I was 15 years old. I lost 2 stone [13 kilos] in weight and used Clomid to aid fertility and subsequently became pregnant, but miscarried very early on. We tried again, but after countless tests, laparoscopies and tablets, still nothing happened. Eventually I was referred to a new and very thorough consultant; it was he who discovered that one of my fallopian tubes was not completely formed. After all the exploratory surgery I had had, I was amazed that it had passed everyone else's notice. Another year's trying and we found that my right ovary performed well, but was attached to a useless tube, and my left ovary was very slow to respond to treatment, but at least the tube was OK. IVF treatment was the next option – the only option.

We started treatment with a nasal spray and injections. My first scan looked disappointing, so despondency set in and I was warned not to get my hopes up, as it looked unlikely that we'd get much further through the programme. Still, we increased the dosage of my drugs and the next scan showed a very different story. At last, 20 first-class eggs were retrieved and then three fertilised embryos were transferred.

A week after the implant, I began to spot quite heavily and I felt ill. I had a blood test and was found to be pregnant. My hormone levels went up and down for the next two weeks, and the day before my six-week scan the hospital phoned to say that my hormone levels had dropped very low and I should expect to start bleeding during the next week.

Counselling was suggested, to which I readily agreed, but the day my counselling started the bleeding ceased and I felt strangely pregnant. A week later I rang the hospital and after some insistence they performed a pregnancy test, and they were clearly staggered when it was still positive. I felt overjoyed at proving them wrong, and then sad because a scan showed no visible foetus. Another pregnancy test confirmed the positive status and the pregnancy was confirmed as ectopic, and the next morning my good fallopian tube, along with my pregnancy, was removed. I wished I was 6 feet under.

I spent six days of torment in hospital with 15- and 16-year-old girls in for abortions. I heard nurses whispering 'Don't tell anyone in here – a lot of them are infertile.'

So here I am, 31, still 'infertile' and still childless. Friends and family are scared to tell me they are pregnant. It's a very lonely feeling. I grieve for my lost children, and nobody can ever understand. I keep myself going with the knowledge that I have frozen embryos in storage – they are my only hope now.

In the meantime I can't have embryos implanted because of problems with irregular bleeding, so it's back into hospital again for a D&C.

My doctor tells me when I can have a baby; it's not my choice. I am forced to do as he says, but something drives me to try again. I feel so bitter that my only good tube was removed – my only chance of becoming pregnant on my own.

Endometriosis

Endometriosis is a painful disease in which tissue identical to the lining of the uterus begins to grow inside the abdomen. Somehow, cells implant on the outside of the uterus, on the ovaries or bowel, and continue to grow just as if they were inside the uterus. Every month these cells bleed, just as they would if they were on the uterine lining, but since the blood cannot escape through the vagina it flows into the pelvic cavity and creates scar tissue. Thus severe menstrual pain, and cramping in teenage girls, can be early signs of endometriosis. It is still uncertain as to how endometriosis first develops. It is even possible that it is a birth defect. Whatever its cause, it plays havoc with the reproductive system, and is painful and tender.

Proper treatment of the less severe forms of endometriosis allows some 70 per cent of sufferers to become pregnant. A woman's level of fertility following more severe forms depends very much on how much damage has been done to the reproductive organs.

About 15 per cent of all women suffer from endometriosis and, in all, 50 per cent of these women will be infertile. Although endometriosis can occur at any age, it is seen most often in women over 30 who have never had children. Equally, as more and more women postpone childbirth in favour of career development, it is expected by the medical profession that infertility due to endometriosis will increase.

There are currently three leading theories about the causal effects of endometriosis on fertility. These are:

1. The body's defence system may recognise the endometrial tissue as a foreign body and thus create antibodies to attack it. These same antibodies are thought to kill sperm.
2. Endometriosis sufferers may have a higher than normal level of a hormone called prostoglandin, which in turn narrows muscular tubes and prevents pick-up of the egg from the ovary.
3. Endometriosis often shortens the second half of the menstrual cycle. If this time becomes too short, then the uterine lining does not have the opportunity to prepare for a fertilised egg; and even if fertilisation does take place, the unprepared uterus will reject the egg as a spontaneous abortion. It is known that nearly 50 per cent of all pregnant women who suffer from endometriosis will abort.

Anon

A year had passed since we had started trying to conceive, so I made an appointment to see our GP. I knew a little about infertility treatments and issues, having worked with several women who had problems. My husband and I visited the GP. He was very understanding and, after initial questioning about timing, he explained what investigations could be done and the timescale. We both underwent preliminary tests for ovulation, sperm counts, etc. When these were normal, I was referred to the hospital's gynaecology department.

On my first out-patient appointment I saw the consultant for about five minutes. He asked a few questions, told me to take folic acid supplements and then told me to go back to my GP's surgery for some more blood tests for ovulation. In the meantime, he would put me on the list for an exploratory laparoscopy. I had further blood tests as a result of returning to my GP (the consultant hadn't contacted him as he'd said he would), and waited for a follow-up appointment from the hospital. The laparoscopy was done as a day case. I had to starve from midnight the day before, go to hospital at about 8am and was allowed home at 1pm.

Despite the conveyor belt surgery, the care was good. The registrar saw me before the operation and explained the procedure and the nurses were good. I was wheeled out of the ward to theatre at 10.15am and returned at 10.35am. I was in pain and was given a painkilling injection – pain relief was my priority. The nurse explained the findings of the operation. They had found patches of endometriosis. I was quite shocked, having had no symptoms. I was able to read my notes; the letter from the consultant to my GP suggested I could have polycystic ovaries and he suggested empirical treatment with Clomiphene to induce ovulation. The operation, however, showed that this wasn't the case and my fallopian tubes were clear.

I knew that treatment for mild endometriosis was controversial in terms of altering the likelihood of pregnancy. When I mentioned this to the registrar at a follow-up appointment, he disregarded it, saying that I wouldn't be considered for further infertility treatment if the endometriosis wasn't treated. He was abrupt and told me all the possible side effects of Danazol drug treatment (masculinisation, weight gain, reduction in breast size, voice deepening, etc.) and the complications of laser treatment (internal bleeding plus the normal risks of general anaesthetic).

I opted for laser treatment. At the pre-op check, I asked the doctor whether it increased the chances of conception. He said it could but that anxiety can play a huge part in preventing conception, so to calm down. Often I have heard this, but how do you focus your attention elsewhere when you desperately want to conceive and can't?

In for the operation, I spent a whole day on the ward before I went to theatre. This was a complete waste of time and NHS money. It even gave time for the hospital chaplain to visit me – I thought I was going to die. The operation went well, but I had a saline drip and was sick. I was told to see my GP in eight weeks, that all the endometriosis had been burned with the laser and I shouldn't suffer any more pain and heavy periods (I'd never had these – he obviously hadn't read my notes).

My GP referred me to another hospital with a specialist infertility clinic. After two months I had heard nothing, so contacted the consultant's secretary to be told I was on the list for IVF – they hadn't even seen me! I was told that once I'd answered a questionnaire about my age, whether I had any children already and if I was on an adoption list, and was accepted for treatment, I would have to wait two to three years. I found this very upsetting – it confirmed I had a major problem which only intervention could help.

Joanna, our next contributor, visited her GP with menstrual problems and was put on the pill. It was a further six years before endometriosis was diagnosed. She was understandably aggrieved by this.

Joanna
I discovered my infertility problem at the age of 21 when I was diagnosed with endometriosis. I am currently having ovulation problems. I came off the pill at 21 and tried to conceive for 15 months. I had suffered a difficult menstrual history since I was 15 and was bluntly told by a gynaecologist that with my history I would be unlikely to conceive.

I was put on the pill because of my menstrual problems, but I feel that GPs should be on the lookout for girls with potential problems instead of blindly putting them on the pill and sweeping the root cause under the carpet in order to get some peace.

In Britain these days the emphasis is more on career and independence for women, so I feel people think that I shouldn't be so involved in wanting children at my age. I think it is crazy that by the time childless couples go through the torment of infertility they are too old to adopt. IVF and other treatments should be available on the NHS. Women need support from day one, not after a few years when it could be too late. I carried out my own research into what endometriosis was and meant – my GP and gynaecologist were quite blunt and didn't hurry to advise me further. I feel a failure and the issue isn't given enough attention. There should be NHS infertility workshops/clinics going over all aspects and solutions.

My feelings have been disbelief, heartache, bitterness and shock. I felt I was being punished but didn't know what for. Each month when my period comes, I feel let down. I lose my temper and my husband tells me to relax, but nevertheless there's always this black cloud of uncertainty that scares me. I'm terrified of living my life in a constant struggle of hope and disappointment.

The feelings of failure and disappointment highlighted by Joanna are not uncommon. Another endometriosis sufferer added her comments.

Joy
My reaction to not conceiving has changed over the months. Initially, I was certain that within six months I would be

proudly announcing to everyone the news that I was pregnant. As the six months came and went, I found each new period more difficult. I would cry a lot and be very tearful. I felt a failure, frustration, disappointment and the ever-increasing feeling that it will never happen to me. I suppose there is a certain amount of grieving going on, but it's not one that others are aware of. Many people close to me know my situation, but apart from one friend who has infertility problems of her own, others just do not know what it is like. I have had so much kind advice. 'Relax and it will happen,' 'Enjoy the time you have on your own,' etc. I know people mean well, but it just doesn't help. Yesterday I began another period and I realise I am now quite resigned to not getting pregnant. I no longer cry when a period starts, but the feeling of disappointment is so intense and the not understanding is hard to bear. Fortunately, my husband is far more relaxed about the situation and very supportive.

One of the frustrations about not getting pregnant is the way it rules your life. I have spent the last 18 months hardly thinking of anything else and most decisions are taken with it in mind; for example, whether or not to go abroad on holiday. If you could turn your hope off like a tap and let go of the desire to have a child, then somehow it would be easier.

Happily, however, the story can have a happy ending, as our next report shows

Julie

After six months of trying to conceive, I consulted my doctor and was told that if nothing had happened in another three months I would be referred to a gynaecologist. Three months later the tests began. David's tests were all fine.

A laparoscopy and dye test confirmed that my tubes were patent [open] but I had endometriosis, the most probable cause of my infertility. I started on a drug called Danazol to stop my periods and hopefully reduce endometriosis. Three months later I started on Clomiphene, as blood tests showed a hormone imbalance and this drug can help ovulation and thus conception.

Progesterone blood tests showed Clomiphene was correcting the hormone imbalance, so I could continue, but after several months it was decided to do another laparoscopy to see if there had been any change in the endometriosis. It was still bad, and to such an extent that IVF was now our only option but we had to fund it ourselves.

At our first appointment we received lots of information and discovered we could start treatment in a couple of months. I commenced a Synorel nasal spray to shut down my natural ovulation so it could be controlled to produce more eggs, and blood was taken to create the culture for the eggs to grow when fertilised. I also began on Perganol injections every morning.

A scan showed that follicles were building up nicely, but the treatment cycle was then aborted because I was in severe danger of hyperstimulation.

We started again the next month, to the point where a scan showed the follicles were ripening and we were fixed up for egg collection, which was performed with light sedation. The pain was horrendous, but we were really pleased that we had 18 eggs. We went home, but I was taken back into hospital in the early hours with severe abdominal pain and nausea and was kept in until embryo transfer that afternoon. I was very upset that only one egg had fertilised. It was implanted and I was sent home.

I felt increasingly unwell for the next two weeks. I had to go for the blood test, then sit and wait for the unit to ring. I was pregnant. I wanted to tell the world, but it was early days yet. They asked to see me to discuss the symptoms I had been suffering, but before I could get there I was admitted with hyperstimulation (not a very common side effect).

From the moment I arrived at the hospital I was being constantly sick. I was put on a drip to prevent dehydration, alternating with another to flush the excess fluid out of my body. Fluid from my ovaries was accumulating in my abdomen and within two weeks my weight went up by 2 stone [13 kilos] and my stomach swelled to 42 inches [105 cm] (a gain of 15 inches [38 cm] in a week). I had to sleep sitting up, as the pain was unbearable and being controlled by Pethidine injections every four hours, along with Stemetil to stop the sickness and daily Heperin to prevent blood clots. (My poor bottom was numb and like tough hide, black and blue.) They considered an operation to drain the fluid but said it could put the baby at risk, so we agreed to continue as we were. (I had the figure of an elephant and the legs to match.) Two weeks later, when the fluid had worked out of my body, I came home but was still in a lot of pain, and by now my weight had dropped to 7½ stone [48 kilos] – normally I am 9 stone [57 kilos].

The sickness continued until I was five months pregnant. I gave up work at six months (having been back only ten weeks) and prepared for the big day, attending parentcraft and relaxation classes. For the last two months I positively bloomed, and apart from being tired I felt really well and enjoyed being pregnant.

Our baby boy, Daniel, was born at 11.26am on 1 June, by elective Caesarean. He is first grade and worth all we went through to have him here.

Pituitary controls

The control centre for reproduction is jointly shared between the hypothalamus and the pituitary gland. They send messages backwards and forwards between themselves to create the perfect environment for conception. Any imbalance in either of these will create havoc with a woman's fertility. The hypothalamus sends hormonal messages to the pituitary, which in turn signals the ovaries. Any form of pressure on the pituitary (cyst, tumour, any type of growth) can cause it to send flawed messages, or often no message at all. Such diagnoses can frequently be handled by treating the cause of pressure and returning the pituitary to its normal state.

Suzanne

We had been married for two years when we decided to start a family. I stopped taking the pill and imagined it would be simple from there. We just took it for granted that we could have children, like most other couples do, but we were not so lucky. After a couple of months my periods had not returned and I was having terrible headaches, so I consulted my GP. She diagnosed stress and told me to give it time. Then my husband had a serious car accident, leaving him with dislodged joints in his spine and depression caused by the trauma – not ideal when you're trying to relax in order to conceive.

My headaches got worse, and still my periods didn't return. My GP was no help at all. Then my employers introduced a health-care plan, and infertility investigations were included in my benefits. I visited a gynaecologist, who did some initial tests but could find nothing wrong. Finally he X-rayed my head. Two days before Christmas he called, telling me that I was booked in for a scan in the New Year, as he had discovered a problem with my pituitary gland. He reassured me that, at this point, he didn't think it was cancer.

After the scan, I was referred to a specialist in London who did further tests and discovered a tumour on my pituitary gland which was effectively stopping it from working. I felt very aggrieved – if my GP had taken note of my symptoms earlier, I could have avoided three years of pain and frustration in trying to conceive.

The London hospital was wonderful, and the operation to remove the tumour went very well. It was nerve-racking waiting six weeks for the results, but worth it to discover that the tumour was benign. Unfortunately it did start to grow back, which meant a course of radiotherapy.

By now all our friends were having babies and we felt very low. Our friends were so happy with their own families that they were insensitive to our pain. I began to avoid babies – it was just too painful to be near them. My husband is naturally very good with children, and I found it heartbreaking to watch him being denied the chance to have his own.

The specialist in London referred us to an infertility unit when we realised that, although my periods had returned, I still wasn't getting pregnant. We were accepted by the infertility unit, and they conducted more tests. Just when we thought it couldn't get any worse, we discovered that my husband had a sperm count so low that there was no chance of us conceiving naturally. We were told that, thanks to a (then) new concept called ICSI, all might not be lost. We were advised that the procedure would cost us around £2,000, plus the drugs. Our regional health authority will pay for a single course of treatment if you hassle them night and day – which I did. I telephoned them constantly until they agreed just to get rid of me.

We went to an open evening at the hospital, where all of the procedures were explained and we were told how ICSI could help people, even those with a low sperm count, since only a single sperm is needed – injected directly into an egg which will hopefully fertilize.

Only a couple of weeks later we were given an appointment to see a specialist. He was very nice and explained that ICSI was our only option and, as with all infertility treatment, the success rate was very low. After seven years we now had funding and an available process which might help, and I couldn't help but feel optimistic.

I used a nasal spray four times each day, to switch off my pituitary gland (I was very reluctant to do this after all that had already happened, but there seemed to be no choice). After a couple of weeks, I returned to the hospital for an internal scan to check that my ovaries had not produced any follicles. This was followed by daily injections to stimulate follicle growth. I was lucky – a local nurse agreed to give the injections (I even went to her home at weekends). When, finally, I had grown enough follicles, the hospital asked me to come in for egg retrieval. I was given a local anaesthetic and the follicles were removed. It was only slightly painful. My husband had to produce a sperm sample (he found this very embarrassing – there is not enough done to help with the comfort and privacy of this procedure: he had to use an empty consulting room, with people walking by and trying the door handle).

We were told that eight eggs had been retrieved and they would call us the next day to let us know if any were successfully fertilised. That night neither of us slept. When the phone rang next morning we could hardly bring ourselves to answer it, but it was OK – four had fertilised and three could be implanted the following Monday. We were on cloud nine – everything had gone so smoothly, we tried not to get too excited, but it was hard not to.

On Monday the embryos were implanted. I was scared to get up afterwards; I had visions of them falling out! We were so careful – my husband wouldn't let me do any housework or lifting.

Almost two weeks after the transplant, it failed and my period arrived. I cannot explain the devastation that I felt. I looked out of my bedroom window and saw the neighbours playing with their children. I really hated them at that moment – I know it sounds horrible, but that's how I felt; it was a mixture of sadness, anger and bitterness. I felt guilty and useless that I couldn't do what everyone around me took for granted.

I dreaded telling my husband, but when he came home I didn't need to say a word; my face was enough. He tried to comfort me, but I knew that he felt as bad as I did. We just sat in the dark all evening, holding each other. We hadn't told anyone else that we had been through the treatment, and I was glad – it was bad enough without having other people's expectations to live up to.

We have had two more attempts since then, both of which we have had to pay for ourselves. Neither has gone as smoothly as the first. Our local clinic has been very supportive and when our last attempt failed, one of the nurses cried with us.

We have now been told that I will have to have my hormone level checked before another attempt, because I don't produce enough follicles even with increased dosage.

We are back at square one, but I know that as long as there is breath left in my body we will keep going. It is a lot to go through – the cost alone can be crippling, but no one thinks that infertility is a just case for the National Health Service. The stress of the treatment is draining, and an understanding employer is vital. But at the end of the day you just can't stop; if there is any hope at all, you just grab hold of it and don't let go. I truly believe, though, that it is important to fill your life with other things as well, so that you don't look back on wasted years spent dreaming of what might have been. I know that the pressure can split couples apart – it is important never to shut each other out, or to keep all the pain within yourself.

Male infertility

A low sperm count in a man can be caused by a multitude of reasons, and often a complete diagnosis will never be made. In terms of a couple's fertility, the only male factor that needs investigation is the sperm count – reasons for the level are, in direct terms, not necessarily relevant, although they can be extremely important to the man concerned.

Realistically, less than 2 per cent of infertile men are actually sterile, which is very good news with the current advances in fertility treatment. In spring 1997 a child was born to a man with azoospermia (zero sperm count), since it is now possible to take a single immature sperm direct from a man's testicles, develop it in a laboratory and then inject it directly into an egg. At the time of writing, two other men are also hoping to become fathers following pioneering operations developed by the gynaecologist Rajat Goswamy at the Churchill Clinic in London. While men with a zero sperm count have no sperm in their seminal fluid, they apparently do have a small amount in their testes. Goswamy's surgery, which takes only ten minutes, involves a small incision to remove a tiny piece of tissue that is then used to fertilise the woman's eggs.

In 1996 the *British Medical Journal* reported that men born in the 1970s could soon have sperm counts up to 25 per cent lower than those of men born in the 1950s. There have been various popular theories to explain the increase in male infertility – these include tight underpants, pesticide poisoning, stress levels and long spells of driving. French research points out that taxi and lorry drivers (along with other drivers covering 25,000 miles [40,000 km] or more a year) are particularly susceptible where the testicles are kept unnaturally warm for long periods of time.

Three possible issues are debated by scientists – increased population density, stress and environmental pollution.

It is known that all animal species have a natural instinct to hold back their numbers when food becomes scarce, and although humans have learned to control their food supplies it is possible that we, too, have a similar innate biological instinct. Perhaps sperm production dips in response to a growing density of population – if so, then it is likely that the direct cause of this response is stress.

Stress is debated everywhere we look, and this book does not endeavour to compete. It is enough to offer the suggestion that if stress can be held part responsible for cancer, heart disease and family breakdown, then it is hard to believe that it cannot cause a drop in fertility.

The toxicity of our environment has also been much debated. Suffice it to say that it is proved beyond doubt that halogenated hydrocarbons, used in both the chemical and petroleum industries, carry a high risk of damage to the reproductive organs. One of the latest suggestions to hit the tabloids is that shampoos and shaving foams, as well as other toiletries containing chemicals, can lower a male sperm count. Spermicides and the inside of condoms are also cited as risky. The chemicals known as alkyl phenol ethoxylates (APEs) are the main chemicals causing concern, as scientists believe that they can be absorbed through the skin. They behave like the female hormone oestrogen, killing off the effectivity of the male hormones.

The Impotence Association also lays the blame for decreasing fertility firmly at the door of cigarette smoking. In addition, there have been suggestions that mothers taking early versions of the contraceptive pill in the 1960s have inadvertently affected the sperm count and motility of their son's sperm.

Sharon

Unfortunately we left trying for a baby until quite late, due to the fact that my husband had been waiting for a kidney transplant for 18 years. We always said we would try for a baby when he had received a transplant. As we were both getting older and we wanted children anyway, we started to try. As nothing was happening, our doctor agreed to a sperm count being done. This came back with a count of zero and it was due to my husband's long-term kidney dialysis.

In February 1995 we found out that it might be possible that there were sperm in the testes and these could be made available and used in IVF. We were referred in April 1995 to see if this was possible. In May 1995 we started with blood tests and during the summer we saw various specialists, including one from London. We applied for funding but were told that this was not available in that financial year.

Fortunately both my husband and I are in full-time employment, so with the house remortgaged we started out on our first attempt at IVF with a testicular biopsy and with ICSI used to fertilise the eggs (one of the first to be done in the Midlands).

Our first attempt produced enough eggs to implant three and freeze four. Between autumn 1995 and spring 1996 we had used all of these up and unfortunately had no luck.

We decided to try again, so I started injecting in April and even though we knew we didn't have as many eggs this time we still went for it. We had enough sperm still left, but again the attempt was unsuccessful. However, we were left with one frozen embryo. During this attempt my local health authority had agreed to fund us, but would not fund any of the £6,500 spent already.

So with a promise of funding we set out at the beginning of this summer to try again. My egg collection produced nine, and then five were successfully fertilised using frozen sperm and ICSI, with three implanted and two frozen (leaving us with three frozen embryos). We are now at the stage where we are waiting again.

I start back to work next week and again it is a waiting game. We have funding from the authority for one more attempt so we will keep trying, but the failure is getting harder to cope with each time.

We are still waiting for a kidney transplant and still trying to have that elusive baby to help us just to be 'normal'!

Hillary and Douglas

My husband and I started trying for a family in 1989, a year after our marriage. After a fruitless year we were referred to the John Radcliffe Hospital in Oxford, where they discovered that my husband had a low sperm count and referred us to a clinic which specialises in male infertility. They gave us two choices – IVF (with a less than 15 per cent chance of success and a cost of approximately £2,000) or IUI (interuterine insemination: about a 20 per cent chance of working and a cost of £125). We opted to try IUI first, but also went immediately onto the IVF waiting list. We still had to wait two years for IUI, and then had seven failed attempts, so we decided to try IVF. Our clinic was now using SUZI with IVF – a procedure where they split the outer coating of the embryo to enable the sperm to reach the inner egg. This procedure had raised our chance of success to 20 per cent.

I began my IVF treatment in June 1994, using a nasal spray twice daily, and once my hormones had reached baseline I commenced Perganol injections. Everything went according to plan and I was admitted for egg recovery. Six eggs were removed, and we were to call the next day to see if any had fertilised. I was told that one egg had been successful, and I was to go in to have it put back. By the time I arrived at the hospital a second egg had fertilised, so two were replaced. I then had to wait the longest two weeks of my life for a pregnancy test. I was convinced that the process had been unsuccessful, but the nurse said she would do the test anyway. She came back five minutes later to say it was positive. I just burst into tears.

Two weeks later a scan showed that I was expecting a single baby. My husband had just changed jobs and was working in the Canary Islands, so at eight weeks pregnant I went to join him there. At 33 weeks gestation I returned to England to await delivery, and my consultant decided not to let me go beyond my due date. Luckily I went into labour naturally, had a normal delivery and Tom was born, weighing 7lb 4oz [3.29kg]. After two weeks we went home to La Palma.

I did not want there to be a big gap in the ages of my children, so we started our second IVF attempt eight months later. The hospital we went to did not do SUZI now, but used ICSI instead – a method of actually injecting one sperm into the middle of the embryo. Again I had six eggs removed, and again two fertilised. This time, though, I went straight back to La Palma and did my own pregnancy test two weeks later. This was negative and a great disappointment to us both, as I think we had both felt that it would work first time as it had before. I think, though, that it was a great help having Tom.

I am currently going through IVF again for our third attempt. If this doesn't work, then for financial reasons we will have to wait longer before we try again, maybe a year or two, although being 34 already I do not feel that time is on our side. I know, though, that I am one of the lucky ones as I have a beautiful little boy who has brought so much joy, not only into the lives of my husband and myself, but also our immediate families as well.

ICSI

It is of interest to note that the Health Council of the Netherlands has called for tighter regulations on the technique known as ICSI, and has requested a moratorium on two specific types of this technique because of fears that it may be risky and lead to abnormal foetal development. The Dutch feel that the technique was introduced without being first properly tested.

ICSI was first successfully tried in Brussels in 1993. Since then approximately 80,000 couples around the world have been treated, resulting in about 20,000 pregnancies. In the United Kingdom it is estimated that around 2,000 children have been born so far as a direct result of ICSI treatment. The two types of technique causing particular concern are MESA (microsurgical epididymal sperm aspiration) and TESE (testicular sperm extraction), where the sperm is removed surgically by a doctor. The fear is that the sperm may not be fully mature, thus increasing the risk of foetal abnormalities. The French government, however, has given permission for 50 specialist centres to begin ICSI treatment.

Research has shown that couples who undertake ICSI are three times more likely to produce a child with certain genetic defects than those who have conceived naturally. A study of nearly 900 children born after their parents had ICSI treatment found that more than 1 per cent suffered defects to their sex chromosomes, which can lead to sterility and mental retardation in later life. This figure compares with less than 0.3 per cent in the general population. Scientists who carried out the study recommend that all couples seeking ICSI treatment are warned of the potential dangers and offered prenatal diagnosis to identify foetuses with defective chromosomes. Dr Maryse Bonduelle, who has led the research team at Brussels Free University, is quoted as saying that it is possible to miss the defects at birth. The signs can be hidden at the beginning, but they often become apparent at puberty.

The reason is believed to be that while, during intercourse, defective sperm cannot normally swim up to the egg cell, ICSI treatment bypasses this natural system for rejecting damaged sperm cells. Researchers believe that the birth defects in the ICSI children are as a result of using defective sperm, rather than due to the treatment itself. It is impossible to test thoroughly the genetic quality of the sperm used without risking further damage.

Derek Tuffnell of Bradford Royal Infirmary feels that there is inevitably a risk in all branches of fertility treatment. He notes too that in addition to the physiological risks, the direct cost of the initial treatment is just the beginning of spiralling costs to infertile couples, the NHS and society as a whole. His hospital has noticed the increasing costs of natal care (since many IVF live births are multiple births, often premature) in line with their infertility activity.

It is too early for the medical profession to know the risks of damage to these 'miracle babies', but there certainly has to be an increased risk of foetal abnormalities with the use of immature sperm. Statistics will not reveal the true nature of this impact, since many such foetal abnormalities will be discovered during the more stringent antenatal checks offered to IVF mothers and will be aborted, thus never registering on statistical analyses.

Ectopic pregnancies

Occasionally a fertilised ovum fails to complete its journey to the uterus; instead it implants in a fallopian tube, or even in the abdominal cavity. This is called an ectopic pregnancy and can be caused by endometriosis, or by a mechanical obstruction within the fallopian tube. The number of reported ectopic pregnancies increased enormously in the 1970s and beyond, and currently the rate is thought to be 1 in 100 pregnancies, caused primarily by higher maternal age and more assisted conception among women with tubal problems.

There is little doubt that the majority of tubal problems are caused by the huge increase in pelvic inflammatory disease (PID). Within the fallopian tubes, PID can cause scarring and obstructions which block the passage of the fertilised ovum to the uterus. Women with a history of tubal infection are seven times more likely than others to have ectopic pregnancies.

In recent years, with the advancement of laser surgery, it is often possible to remove the embryo without damaging the tube or the ovary. In cases where the ectopic pregnancy has been caused by an obstruction in the fallopian tube there is inevitably a high risk of another ectopic pregnancy, unless the tube is in some way reconstructed. Newer methods of treating ectopics include laparoscopy where potassium chloride can be injected to destroy the pregnancy. This is beneficial if the ectopic is diagnosed early enough, but little can be done to save the tube after it has burst. One (currently experimental) procedure is that of relocation – removing the pregnancy and replacing it in the uterus. Success has, so far, been limited but at least work is being done in this important area.

Alexandra and David started trying for their second baby when their son, Charles, was one.

Alexandra
Nothing happened, and after a couple of years, we realised something must be wrong.

With the help of fertility drugs, Alexandra finally got pregnant. She was overjoyed. But eight weeks later, a scan revealed that the baby was growing in her fallopian tube instead of in her womb. The tube had to be removed, bringing the pregnancy to an end. 'We felt dreadful', she remembered. 'But we thought at least I still had another tube; we still had a chance of another baby.'

Two years later Alexandra was pregnant again, but this time her joy was mingled with fear. Then fate dealt another cruel blow – the baby was growing in her only remaining fallopian tube. She had to have another operation – and with the second operation, all the couple's hopes of a second child died. 'I was absolutely devastated,' said Alexandra. For a long time the couple couldn't bear to think about having more infertility treatment. But they were still desperate to have another baby. And their first son, Charles, was desperate to have a brother.

'He couldn't understand why he didn't have any brothers,' Alexandra recalled. 'He used to ask me why he couldn't have one, and it was hard to know what to say.'

The couple bravely decided to pay for IVF treatment and to have aftercare through the NHS. Eggs were extracted from Alexandra's body and fertilised with David's sperm, then implanted in her womb.

'The treatment worked first time,' said Alexandra. 'I was so lucky; many couples have to try over and over again.'

The couple were delighted to find they were going to have twins. Staff at the hospital monitored the pregnancy carefully, giving the couple comfort and support every step of the way. But 16 weeks on, tragedy struck again. A scan revealed that one of the babies had died.

> We couldn't believe it. We thought that after all we'd been through, we were going to lose both babies. The staff were wonderful with us. I had several tests to check on the progress of my remaining baby. I was so worried. I think I might have lost him had it not been for all the help and support the staff gave us.

When little Oliver was born on 16 October, he was normal apart from two minor problems which can be corrected – his tiny feet turned inwards and he had a kidney complaint. Now splints have been strapped to his legs to straighten his feet, and he is making good progress. Alexandra said:

> I still cry sometimes when I hold him in my arms. I still can't believe he's here. All I seem to have read about this hospital and the NHS in general are complaints. But I have nothing but praise for the hospital and its staff.

Non-specific tubal blockages

Debbie
My husband and I married when I was 32 and after six months of marriage decided that, mainly because of my age, we should

start our family. I duly came off the pill and happily looked forward to a pregnancy.

After six months I was a little worried and visited my GP, who prescribed a fertility drug (Clomid, I think), and ovulation tables and thermometers – all very romantic! Still nothing. I trotted back to the doctor, who arranged for me to go and have dye injected through my tubes to check for blockages.

I was told there was a problem, so I visited a consultant, who arranged for me to go in for a laparoscopy. I was admitted to a small two-bed ward, along with a woman who was in for a sterilisation, which I found a little ironic. I must say that for each of my appointments I had to walk through the antenatal clinic and labour ward in order to get to the infertility clinic. I realise various equipment is shared, but I still feel that the layout of the hospital is very insensitive to people like me.

The result of the laparoscopy was conclusive. My fallopian tubes were totally blocked, with no chance of successful treatment. Up until this point I had remained positive, but finally it hit home – if I wanted a baby I was going to have to fight for it. I was put on the NHS waiting list for IVF treatment, but was told it was 18 months long, which seemed like an eternity away, with my body clock ticking louder every month.

My husband supported me, but has never had the yearning for a child that I have felt since I was a young woman. I always envisaged having a loving family around me and a feeling of fulfilment and normality.

Anyway, we decided to go to a private clinic for a consultation on IVF. They accepted our case and we both underwent various tests to begin with. The clinic was about half an hour's drive from our home, so I arranged to have the daily injections required at the local doctor's surgery during the week, and at the clinic at weekends. As I had to have these injections for about six weeks, it became quite a routine (and a bit of a pain), but I pushed myself on, knowing it would be worth it in the end. Financially, we didn't have much in the way of savings (being fairly newly married), so my mother-in-law kindly gave us £1,500 to pay for the initial treatment.

At last the time arrived for egg collection. The procedure took place without anaesthetic, just a dose of Pethidine which had no effect, so the event was fairly painful.

My husband produced a sperm sample to fertilise the eggs. Fourteen eggs were retrieved, eleven of which were good so, two days later, three fertilised eggs were replaced in my womb and the wait began. The spare fertilised eggs were frozen for future use.

Two weeks later I had a pregnancy test which was negative. I was shattered, although I knew I had at least two more attempts with the remaining eggs. After a few months we tried again, using three more eggs which had been defrosted, and the same thing happened.

I can remember sitting in the clinic, full of pictures of babies born after successful treatment, and crying when the nurse told me the result. Still, I had some frozen eggs left which we decided to use after a few more months of saving up (a cost of £400–500 each treatment). I was pinning all my hopes on this last attempt and psyched myself up for the course of injections and preparations.

But luck wasn't on my side and my hopes were dashed again.

In the back of my mind I knew I was still on the NHS waiting list and was told, after I had telephoned to enquire how I was getting along on the list, to phone again in six months time.

I was finally called for treatment after another three years. I had a feeling that everything was going to work out with the NHS, and began to feel optimistic. I started my treatment and got so far into the injections and went for a scan to check progress. Unfortunately it was discovered that my ovaries were being overstimulated and the treatment had to stop. I fell into work and cried on the shoulder of a friend there. I was sent home in a dreadful state.

The treatment was started again shortly afterwards. This time I had egg retrieval under general anaesthetic and eight good eggs were collected. Unfortunately they had no facility to freeze unused eggs at the NHS hospital, so it was a case of one chance with three eggs. I had these implanted two days later and started waiting again – every day seemed to last forever, dreading going to the loo in case I had started to bleed.

On the tenth day the bleeding started, so I knew that was it. I spent the rest of the day in a trance trying to come to terms with the fact that I was never going to be a mother.

We had decided not to persevere any more as I was 39 and we thought I had been through enough both emotionally and physically. I still find it very difficult to cope with. Friends are having babies all the time and I still find it hard to envisage life without children, but I've recently celebrated my 40th birthday and realise that I have got to go forwards and believe I gave it my best shot.

I will now concentrate on other things in life. I have a super husband and we share a good life together which we will enjoy to the full, albeit with a constant sadness in my heart.

4 IVF and its successes

The IVF technique pioneered in the 1970s by Steptoe and Edwards was developed originally to treat patients who have blocked or damaged fallopian tubes (so that the sperm and egg cannot meet), but as it has become more successful it has been used to treat a much wider spectrum of infertility disorders. To obtain a reasonable success rate with IVF more than one egg needs to be collected during the treatment cycle. This is achieved by using fertility drugs.

The first principle of the treatment is to stop the body's normal control mechanisms for ovulation. To do this a type of medication known as a gonadatrophin releasing hormone agonist (GNRH agonist) will typically be used. There are different forms of this drug which can be administered daily as a nasal spray (for example, Nafarelin and Buserelin), by subcutaneous injection (Buserelin), or by a subcutaneous injection that lasts for four weeks (Zoladex and Prostap). The drug most commonly employed is Nafarelin nasal spray. This step in the treatment is important as it makes the process a lot simpler, it allows the consultant to plan the cycle more readily and, finally, it does appear substantially to increase the success of the treatment. Having stopped the body producing its own hormones, those necessary for the production of mature eggs can then be administered medically. These hormones are collectively called human menopausal gonadotrophins (HMG). As the name would suggest, they are derived from the urine of postmenopausal women and are therefore natural hormones. The common brand names include Perganol, Humegon, Normegon, Orgafol and Metrodin HP. For the purposes of IVF all these medications act in a similar fashion and are interchangeable.

The development of the follicles containing the eggs is monitored indirectly through blood tests and directly by visualising the ovary using a vaginal ultrasound probe.

When mature, the eggs are collected using the same vaginal ultrasound probe with an attached guided needle. The eggs are placed in test tubes in culture fluid. On the morning of the egg collection the man produces a sperm sample by masturbation. The best sperm are then selected using a sperm wash technique and after six hours are added to the test tubes containing the eggs. The following morning the eggs are inspected for signs of fertilisation. If fertilisation has occurred the early embryos are transferred to the uterus 48 hours after the eggs were collected. A maximum of three embryos are transferred through the cervix into the uterus using a soft catheter. A sensitive pregnancy test is performed 14 days after the egg collection to confirm a pregnancy.

Despite considerable advances in recent years, IVF remains a complex and expensive treatment. Just over one in every five patients will have a successful pregnancy after one cycle of IVF treatment. The chance of a successful treatment cycle does depend to some extent on the reason why the patient cannot conceive naturally, and on the patient's age.

Studies have shown that just over 55 per cent of women under the age of 34 will conceive after completing five treatment cycles of IVF.

Samantha

I haven't been given a cause for my infertility except that I once had endometriosis, but was treated and told that was clear. We have had four private IVF attempts. Infertility treatment should be freely available on the NHS. IVF is very expensive and it seems as if you have to have money to have a child. It took us a long time to save for each treatment, which prolonged the process when we weren't getting any younger.

IVF is very stressful. I felt like an egg machine trying to make as many eggs as I could. It just seemed to be drugs, injections and blood tests. Before starting treatment I was very anxious but at the same time positive, which I think is a good feeling to have. During the treatment, I was awful to live with – really snappy and with terrible mood swings. It was good that we had a strong relationship. I can understand people splitting up during treatment. It is very hard for both the man and the woman. After treatment I felt like a walking timebomb, waiting to see if I was pregnant or not, waiting to see if I was going to bleed. Every time you go to the toilet you expect to see something you do not want to. I was also scared in case something I did would stop it from working. The IVF treatment did not affect my general life, except that you do wonder if you are ever going to have a child and then you do have days when you feel very down. In the beginning we considered adoption but were told that we were too old, so as well as IVF we thought we would try fostering which we were given the OK for. The first IVF treatment gave us our little girl and then we considered fostering, but then our final IVF resulted in twin boys so our family is now complete.

In hindsight, I don't think my fertility problems were investigated enough. I didn't really think about it at the time – it was only later when a friend had many more investigations done that I wondered. Although it was private treatment, it all seemed too clinical and we felt as though we were purely there to fund their research, although the nursing staff were very professional and always at the end of the phone if needed. Our failed attempts met little sympathy, though we were offered the help of a counsellor which we declined.

There is a stigma attached to infertility – and to the treatment, come to that. I assume the ignorant parties are those that can have children easily and without having to have treatment. They seem to come across as not caring and thinking that a lot of fuss is being made over nothing. I can see the future of infertility treatment going a long way – it will get better and better and a lot more people who couldn't have children will have them, but if the cost continues to rise, it will only be for those that can afford it.

My only comment to those who are trying IVF or some other treatment is: don't give up, be patient and optimistic. I got the impression that because I had children through IVF, I should always be happy. We paid a lot of money out and went through a lot to have them, so people tended to think that I should always have a smile on my face. It can be very hard work with my one-year-old twin boys and a four-year-old girl. We are very grateful for IVF treatment and know that without it, we could still now be trying to conceive naturally.

Many of those contributors lucky enough to end up giving birth following infertility treatment encounter difficulties along the way.

Pru and Mark

I have damaged fallopian tubes apparently caused by PID following an infection, chlamydia. I have never had any symptoms of either, or any reason to believe that I have had an infection. I haven't had any casual sexual partners and I have no idea how they got damaged. I did have my gall bladder removed at the age of 19 but doctors seem to think it very unlikely that this had anything to do with it.

Pru explained her feelings about being childless before her private IVF treatment:

I never imagined my life without a family and when it became clear that having a baby wasn't going to be easy, it absolutely devastated me – I was panicked, shocked and distraught. I never believed I would be one who had trouble. Now I have a son, Oliver, as a result of IVF. Before the treatment I felt almost excited – at least we were getting on with it. During treatment I got a bit fed up with the nasal spray and the whole thing went on for so much longer as we had a cancelled cycle due to over-stimulation which really depressed me; I felt as if I couldn't do anything right, as cancelled cycles only happen apparently around 5 per cent of the time. During treatment I became a lot worse about seeing babies and pregnant people. I was always thinking, 'I wonder how many were conceived with fertility treatment.' It also really upset me to see young mothers of large families screaming at their kids – everything seemed so unfair.

When we had the embryos put back I felt more positive and optimistic. The positive pregnancy test was an obvious joy but it wasn't until after twelve weeks that I relaxed a bit and not until Oliver was born that I relaxed more. The process has made me more understanding and I realise that I can't have everything I want – my life had been pretty trouble-free and most things came quite easily to me: infertility was my burst bubble. Also, I am convinced that I appreciate my baby so much more than if I hadn't had problems.

Pru also suffered ectopic pregnancy.

After our first ectopic pregnancy (loss of a tube and told the other one was also damaged), no one seemed to have any sympathy at all and the doctors explained the situation very badly. It was only after one of the hospital doctors saw how upset I was that he suggested an appointment with the consultant within two weeks. When this didn't happen, I rang the hospital and spoke to the consultant's NHS secretary who told me he had nothing available for three to four months. Luckily we had private insurance, so I rang his private secretary (who was very supportive and understanding) and we had an appointment within two weeks. From then on, the only counselling we had was at the fertility centre whose counsellor was very, very helpful. It was effectively five to six months after the first devastating news of my infertility that I could get everything off my chest.

Pru explained her feelings:

People who have no problems don't recognise it properly or realise what is involved. Unless you tell people, no one suspects. When you do tell them, most people think the general public need to be made much more aware of infertility and how damaging emotionally it can be for those involved. Unfortunately, whenever something goes wrong, the press have a field day and the old questions crop up again. The very fertile majority have no idea what it is like to have problems. At my coffee morning group (mums and babies) we were discussing the Mandy Allwood case [see Chapter 1] and how she was told not to have sex during her treatment. One woman said, 'they really should think about who they give this treatment to when there are so many unwanted children in this country.' People who make these types of comments, together with the many who don't believe fertility treatment should be available on the NHS, have no idea what is involved.

Finally, Pru was damning of her own GP's attitude:

My original GP refused to fund anything to do with the treatment, so I rang the local health authority to give me a list of GPs who would fund the drugs – the list was limited and my new GP could only fund the drugs for one cycle (which is better than nothing). If I had lived somewhere else, I might even have got the whole treatment on the NHS – it seems unfair that your treatment is decided just because of where you live. If we didn't have the money to fund our own treatment, we would still be without a pregnancy.

Regarding other complications, the Leeds General Infirmary's Assisted Conception Unit provides the following comments.

There are two main complications that can occur with IVF treatment – hyperstimulation and multiple pregnancies. These both arise because of the need to use infertility drugs to produce a group of mature eggs that will give you a better chance of a pregnancy.

Hyperstimulation is where the ovaries over-respond to the hormone injections used to stimulate the growth of the eggs. Rather than the usual number of around ten eggs, many eggs may start to mature. This can result in the ovaries enlarging, with some abdominal discomfort. The very high concentrations of hormones made by these developing eggs can make the patient feel nauseous. Very rarely fluid can accumulate in the abdomen due to the large hormone producing ovaries. This can thicken the blood, making the kidneys less efficient and the blood more likely to clot. Thankfully these problems are rare, and if managed carefully should not cause any long-term problems. Precautions are taken to ensure that the risk of hyperstimulation is small.

In the case of multiple pregnancies, it is obvious that if more than one embryo is replaced in the uterus there is a chance that the patient may have more than one baby. Most people would not mind twins, though they might be concerned by triplets, but there are potentially serious implications involved in any multiple pregnancy: a greater risk of miscarriage, premature delivery (with the possible death or handicap of one or all babies) and the necessity for the babies to spend some time on the special care baby (intensive care) unit. There is also an increased chance of spending time in hospital with problems such as raised blood pressure or other medical conditions during the pregnancy, and an increased chance of needing a Caesarean section to deliver the babies. Finally, when she gets her babies home the new mother may well need some assistance to help the family to cope.

Most fertility units will never replace more than three embryos per treatment, acting according to HFEA guidelines, although there is no legal limit. And in certain circumstances where it is felt that the risk of a triplet pregnancy is high, then only two embryos are replaced. This is routine in patients under 35 years of age. There are guidelines which can be used to assess the risk of triplets in any particular couple.

Carol is the mother of Charlotte, Luke and Gary, her IVF triplets.

Carol

I got married and later stopped taking the pill. After six to nine months nothing had happened and the GP told us to try for longer. We then moved area and changed GP. After seeing this GP we had been trying for 18 months and were referred to our local hospital. I had blood tests to check I was ovulating. I was. A laparoscopy and D&C were carried out which showed blocked tubes – one totally and one partially. It took three months for the unblocking procedures and a six-month try to get pregnant. I was transferred to a specialist hospital for IVF. There was a three-year waiting list on the NHS and we were allowed three attempts, but if we had one done privately, then we would 'lose' one NHS attempt.

I got pregnant naturally after two years, but at six to seven weeks it was found to be ectopic. We went to a lecture on IVF, then had an assessment. I had blood tests for AIDS etc. and was given a date to start treatment. I'd always assumed I'd stop taking the pill and get pregnant – I don't like hospitals or injections and thought, 'Why me?' My tubes were apparently blocked because of pelvic infection and I was angry I'd taken the pill for years when I didn't need to. More should be done really before the pill is prescribed, like a simple scan.

I had to phone the hospital on day one of my period to see if there was an available place – there wasn't, so I couldn't start the treatment. It was agreed with my GP to give me the drugs needed so I could start with my next period. On the first day I had a blood test and an internal scan (slightly uncomfortable, like a smear test). Then started injections in my arm, which my GP did. After seven days I was back at the hospital. If my hormone level was down, I could start the second lot in my bum for ten days. My follicles weren't of good enough size and my hormone levels were not high enough so the treatment was abandoned, but it doesn't count as a treatment unless it gets as far as egg replacement.

I found myself going twice a day to the hospital. On the second attempt I got seven eggs, three of which fertilised. The eggs were replaced and I stayed at the hospital for eight hours. I had another injection and had to wait for my period – or not. I felt generally unwell (I hadn't felt 100 per cent since having my tube removed with the ectopic) and in quite severe pain. I got my period and was really upset. Now I wish they'd abandoned it earlier. My husband, Gary, simply said, 'Well, it hasn't worked; let's try again. Crying won't help.' I thought he was heartless.

I still get upset about my ectopic, even now. Luckily I kept my ovary afterwards – it could have been a total hysterectomy. I should have had three more periods before trying again, but it turned into a six-to-seven-month wait as there were no places. The first time, I was full of hope. I hadn't even told my Mum the second time. I never went to the GP – I didn't want anyone to know. Telling people it hadn't worked first time was hard – friends were ringing, customers where I worked asked about it; it all added to the trauma. I didn't want to tell the world and its wife. I felt it very personally.

The next time, I had a higher dosage of drugs and felt much better – all went well. I produced eleven or twelve follicles, but all the follicles were empty. Apparently, the same happened to someone else and it was thought to be due to a faulty batch of HCG. I was devastated. There followed another three-month break to get the drugs out of my system. Then back to the hospital. I was left on a higher dosage and responded as I should – eight follicles, eight eggs. Eight fertilised but one fertilised with two sperm so wasn't used. Four were frozen and three were implanted. We could use, donate or destroy the frozen ones later.

The frozen egg issue now bothers me – genetically, they are mine; potentially, they are my children's brothers or sisters. What happens if they meet up later? I'd like to donate them because I've met people who can't produce eggs, but now I'm unsure. Gary thinks it is selfish not to donate but he'll stand by my decision. The hospital asked me about my eggs at the beginning but I've heard nothing since and the time limit is nearly up.

At the assessment, I was told they will take women up to 40, and you can have anything wrong other than AIDS. There was no support available though when it failed (like with my ectopic). It didn't really put a strain on us but we had other interests – I went to the gym and he went to football. It does consume your life for a few weeks and you wonder what you'll do when the treatment finishes. For us, it was just something we had to do and we did it. I was a bit obsessed – it was something I wanted, but I still led a normal life. The problems might have come if we'd been told it couldn't work, but there was always light at the end of the tunnel. On days when I freaked out, Gary ignored it and let it all ride over him. I was rampaging and he was very laid back.

Nothing would have stopped me; I'd have tried anything. Once IVF was out of the question, I'd have thought about adoption. I still tend to stare at newborn babies; it makes me feel jealous and broody even now. We'd tried for seven years so it is hard to give up that yearning. It's really selfish – I just want to sit and nurse a newborn baby all day.

Anyway, last attempt – three eggs were replaced and I lay in bed for eight hours talking to three eggs, telling them how much I wanted them to stay where they were. It's a good job I was in a room by myself. Back for the pregnancy test – I was pregnant! Back for a scan in six weeks. Very early on I was sick all day. By the third week, I rang the hospital who said it could be more than one. I was sick every day, vomiting. I had to go to hospital with a bucket, I was so bad. I lost a stone [6.5 kilos] in two weeks. I sat in the hospital corridor with my head between my legs. They did an internal scan because I couldn't keep a jug of water down, and found three heartbeats. Gary was there – the nurse said she didn't know who looked worse, Gary or me.

The pregnancy was fine, but all through I was told I was in a high-risk group for miscarriage and worried all the time that something would happen. The sickness was the only bother I had. At 18 weeks I was put on steroid injections to develop their lungs in case I went into early labour, but my cervix was always closed and the babies were a good size. I went from 9 to 16 stone [57 to 101 kilos]. They were born at 35 weeks – the deliveries were by section with an epidural. I developed arthritis in my spine due to the excess weight, which has been the main problem of carrying triplets.

For those contemplating IVF, I'd say definitely, go ahead. It's hard and you have to dedicate a lot of time to it. There are results for some people. If you don't do it, you'd always wonder if it would have worked. If you don't try, you don't know, but your heart must be in it. And if you do eventually find you are expecting more than one baby, feel lucky but also always ask for help – it is there if you ask for it – you don't realise how much help you will need, so accept all the help you can get.

Helen is one of the very lucky women who found success with her first treatment – she has some valuable points to make.

Helen

I have had extremely painful periods since my teens, often missing school and later work. I was unfortunate in my GP who told me it was normal. My husband and I began trying for a family in 1989 when I was 29. Twelve months on, we had no success. Tests followed and endometriosis was diagnosed. Nine months of treatment followed, with awful side effects. Then a second laparoscopy found there was no improvement and I was told IVF was my only hope of having a baby. I was devastated.

We knew the NHS waiting list was long and couldn't wait, so went privately at a cost of £2,500. Fortunately the treatment was successful on our first attempt, and although I had an awful pregnancy we are now the very proud parents of a two-year-old. Every time I look at him, I am overwhelmed by the miracle of it all – being childless was so awful for me.

The IVF treatment was good, although expensive, and we have been unable to afford it since even though I'd like to try again, but I do appreciate what I've got. I would have done anything if it would have helped, although I remember a lot of prejudice at the time (usually from those who had never experienced childlessness). I often feel so sad that the problems of infertility are not spoken about by couples and I get furious that endometriosis is practically an unknown word.

In some cases there is either no problem or only limited problems with the female reproductive cycle, but natural conception is unsuccessful. In such cases, natural cycle IVF – a treatment somewhat less invasive than full IVF – can be used. Leeds General Infirmary provided us with the following information:

Natural cycle IVF

This refers to the process whereby the eggs produced in a female's normal cycle will be collected, fertilised with a sample of the partner's sperm, and if the egg fertilises the small embryo will be replaced through the cervix some two days later.

At the start, growth of the follicle containing the egg will be monitored by ultrasound scans and blood tests. The potential parents will probably need to attend four to five times during each cycle of treatment. When the follicle containing the egg appears mature, as judged by the scans and blood tests, the donor female will be given an injection of a hormone called human chorionic gonadotrophin (HCG) 5000iu. This acts like the LH hormone, in that it initiates the final maturation processes which lead to ovulation. We aim to collect the egg just before ovulation. The egg collection will involve a vaginal ultrasound probe with a guided needle. The ovaries normally lie very close to the top of the vagina. The needle is inserted, guided by the ultrasound picture, through the vagina and into the ovary. The fluid in the follicle is drained and examined to find the egg. Unfortunately, for a number of reasons, there is no guarantee that an egg will be recovered, even in the presence of a large mature follicle. However, in over 90 per cent of cases the egg collection will be successful.

The egg will be taken to the laboratory, where it will be mixed with a prepared sample of sperm, which will have been produced earlier the same day by masturbation. If the egg fertilises (which occurs in 85 per cent of cases) the small embryo will be replaced in the uterus after 48 hours. In the remaining 15 per cent of cases the egg will either not fertilise or more than one sperm will enter. Should either of these instances occur, there will be no embryo to transfer. The embryo is transferred using a small catheter inserted gently through the cervix into the uterus. This is a relatively painless procedure, similar to having a cervical smear taken.

A blood test 14 days after egg collection will provide evidence of conception. The whole process may be repeated on a monthly basis up to a maximum of three months. The overall chance of achieving a clinical pregnancy is 11.5 per cent per egg collection, although the rate does vary according to the reason treatment is required.

John and Jane, our next contributors, could probably have used natural cycle IVF, but may have decided against it on the basis that full IVF would lead to the implantation of up to three embryos, thus increasing the chance of pregnancy.

John and Jane

March 1985 and John's visit to the family doctor revealed some very swollen glands. After two or three weeks of tests, Hodgkins Disease, Stage 3b was diagnosed.

Acting on advice, John donated some sperm to the Embryology Department at Southampton General Hospital before starting a six-month chemotherapy course. He was warned at the time that the donation could well be of highly inferior quality, heavily affected by the lymphoma. However, the result was frozen anyway. It was not until 1991 (having married in 1988) that John and Jane decided to undergo a course of IVF, hoping to use John's donation. After Jane's drug preparation some sperm straws were thawed out (their quality was not promising). Three embryos were subsequently successfully fertilised with donor sperm, and two with John's. John's were replaced, and after a somewhat anxious wait pregnancy was confirmed around Christmastime 1991.

Thomas Paul was born on 11 September and weighed 5lb 14oz (2.67 kilos). Jane continued:

IVF was tried for a second time towards the end of 1995. (It took time to save, and pluck up courage to have another go.) The plan was to use John's sperm if possible (without donor back-up this time), so back we went to the freezer, and this time two eggs were successfully fertilised. They were both replaced and on 9 July 1996, again after a short labour, James William was born in an ambulance on the hard shoulder of the M5 between Junctions 20 and 19 on the way to the hospital. He weighed 7lb 3oz [3.26 kilos] and was a week early.

We know we are extremely lucky. It is certainly one thing to be cured of Hodgkins, but then to go on to father two healthy children must be considered somewhat of a minor miracle.

We are both very keen to use our story as encouragement to others, even though we have not obviously been through the heartache of an unsuccessful IVF attempt.

Valerie, our last contributor in this chapter, does not just bear witness to IVF programmes, but has also experienced frozen embryo transfer, a controversial process which is in fairly common use today. First, Leeds General Infirmary's Assisted Conception Unit provides the following commentary on the issue of frozen embryo transfer:

> It has been possible for some time to freeze (cryopreserve) embryos which are not used during a full IVF attempt. These embryos can be thawed at a later date and transferred back to the womb after suitable preparation of the lining of the womb in order to receive the embryos.
>
> Transfer of these frozen/thawed embryos is not as successful at establishing pregnancies as the transfer of embryos which have not been frozen, but they do represent a second or even third chance to achieve a pregnancy without having to undergo the full course of injections to stimulate the ovaries and the egg recovery procedure. At the moment evidence suggests the embryos withstand the freezing process better if they are frozen in the very early stages of their development, usually just after fertilisation has been confirmed. This causes a slight problem in that it is important to get two or three good embryos for transfer and it is not known if an embryo is good until it has been allowed to grow for two days. To overcome this, therefore, Leeds allows five embryos to develop and freezes all fertilised eggs in excess of five, providing, of course, the donors request this. This generally ensures that at least three good-quality embryos are available for transfer in the first stimulated cycle of treatment.
>
> Transfer of the frozen embryos can be arranged at any point after the initial full IVF treatment. There is no evidence that embryos are actually affected by the length of time they are frozen. It is understood that any damage is caused during the course of cooling embryos to freezing point and warming to body temperature. Thus it has been known for a couple to achieve two pregnancies from one cycle of treatment and for a couple to have their 'twins' two, three or four years apart.

Valerie

After unsuccessfully trying for a baby for nearly five years, we were referred to the IVF unit at Bristol. This we felt was a massive step forward as until then we had had various tests, none of which shed any light on why I had not yet become pregnant. I had already had various courses of tablets, injections and scans that only resulted in my having two operations, the first a laparoscopy to check my tubes and the second to remove a cyst from one of my ovaries. This was spotted during the laparoscopy.

The consultation was wonderful. This was the first doctor to say that we had been trying long enough for our family and that they could help. Up until this point we had constantly been told that we just had to be patient, or worse still to try to accept that we might never have children. Prior to seeing this consultant I had already undergone about a month of tests down at Bristol. At its peak we were travelling down almost every morning before going to work so that I could be scanned throughout a 'typical cycle' so that they would have some idea as to what my body was doing. This was a round trip of about 100 miles [160 km], all before 8.30 in the morning. Although this was tiring, it meant that by the time we saw the professor he was able to offer us the chance of trying IVF if we wanted to. Of course we said YES.

The treatment started within the week, first with the inhaler, then with the injections. I had a brilliant local surgery where the nurses would fit me in for my injections regardless of how busy they were. Scans followed, more injections followed that, until the day came when my eggs were ready for collection. I had lots of eggs, probably more than they would have liked and had bordered on the safety cut-off point all the way along my treatment. They collected 23 eggs, then we had to wait a couple of days to see if any fertilised – 18 did! We had entered into IVF treatment expecting it to fail at some point. This would then have told us why I could not get pregnant. We were amazed everything had gone so well.

I had three eggs replaced and then had to wait a couple of weeks to see if they would implant. The remaining eggs were frozen in case we decided to try again at a later date. I had intended to have just a couple of days off work and then go back and carry on as normal. Unfortunately I became rather ill within a few days of my egg collection and this was not possible. I had been warned that I might have a delayed reaction to the drugs I had been taking because of having so many eggs on my ovaries. I had been very sick and had to be admitted to hospital where I was put on a drip as I had dehydrated. I had hyper-stimulated as a result of the drugs and within a couple of days my whole body swelled up. It was very painful. It was quite scary and to top it all I didn't even know if I would be pregnant at the end of all this.

After a few days I was well enough to go home, although I was still very swollen and still in quite a bit of pain. I ended up having to take eight weeks off work. By this time I had returned to a normal shape. The good news from all this was that after two weeks I found myself pregnant. I could hardly believe it. Somehow the pain became bearable then. Further scans revealed that I was expecting just one baby. I was so relieved, not at all disappointed that it wasn't twins or triplets. I still had to have injections for the first twelve weeks of pregnancy to help maintain the pregnancy. I must say that I felt like a pin cushion by the end of it all.

I went back to work feeling wonderful, then at eleven weeks I started bleeding. I was horrified and so scared. It was a Friday. The hospital advised us to stay put and for me just to take it easy, then on Monday to go down and have a scan to see if the baby was still there. It was the worst weekend ever. We travelled almost in silence, I think both of us thought we had lost the baby. The hospital staff rushed us through on our arrival and quickly scanned my tummy. Yes, the baby was still there. What a relief!

I spent the first six months of pregnancy bleeding on and off, and at no time was any diagnosis made as to why this was happening. The reason only came to light in my 39th week when I bled again. I was scanned at the maternity hospital. It revealed placenta praevia, which meant that I wouldn't be able to deliver normally, so the next day I had a section and to our great relief Daniel arrived, the picture of health.

When I look back at all the things that nearly did go wrong, I still consider us exceptionally lucky to now have our five-year-old. To be successful on our first IVF attempt was incredible. The odds were not in our favour. I have to say that all the tears and the heartache and the pain were worth it.

Our families were brilliant all the way through the traumatic nine months. They were very supportive and much relieved when Daniel finally arrived. So it probably came as quite a shock when two years later we told them that we were going to try again for number two. I had two attempts with the frozen embryos. The medication was less invasive but the success rate much lower. Both attempts failed. Now if we wanted to try again it would mean full IVF treatment. It was a big decision for me, as I had been so ill the first time. I had no desire to go through that again, especially now that we had Daniel. The staff at

Bristol assured me that it wouldn't happen again and that this time only half the dosage would be used, but this would also mean that I would probably have fewer eggs to collect and therefore fewer to fertilise. We decided to have one last go. Our parents thought we were mad. I think they saw it as such a risk. We had been so lucky first time round and I had been so ill. They supported our decision none the less. The treatment was exactly the same, but this time we knew what to expect at each stage. Everything went along smoothly as before. I had eleven eggs collected this time and of these just three fertilised.

We felt a little disappointed, but then again I felt so much better. I had the three eggs replaced and then we just had to play the waiting game again. This time, though, I just knew I was pregnant. The test confirmed it. We were thrilled to bits. Again the scan showed there was just one baby – once again I was very relieved.

This time the pregnancy was very straightforward. No problems at all and nine months later Adam was delivered normally, two weeks late. He was, and still is, beautiful, just like his brother. He is two years old now.

That's it now. No more IVF. We have been incredibly lucky. I still look at my two and can hardly believe that they are mine.

It makes me so cross to hear people saying that IVF is wrong. That it's interfering with nature. The criticism seems to come from people who either don't want children or who have babies easily. How could anyone look at my boys and tell me what we did was wrong? These people have no idea of what it's like to want a baby so badly, only to find that it seems to be an impossible dream.

I have only praise for the medical staff. They were very supportive throughout and would always find time to explain what was happening. We recently attended a party to celebrate the birth of the 750th IVF baby at the unit. It was a lovely day and we were very happy to be part of it.

5 IVF – when it fails

In terms of success rates for IVF treatment, the most important statistic is the number of women who actually take home one (or more) babies per treatment cycle started. This is officially recorded as the maternity rate (MR) per treatment cycle.

The statistics in Table 4.1 emerged from the Assisted Conception Unit at Leeds General Infirmary. These figures do not take into account any additional pregnancies that occur as a result of the transfer of frozen embryos.

Table 4.1 Maternity rate per treatment cycle, 1991/2 to 1994/5

Year	No. of treatment cycles	Maternity rate
1991/2	251	23.1%
1992/3	373	22.7%
1993/4	643	22.4%
1994/5	738	23.3%

Mandy
I have ovulatory problems, and so far have received two NHS IUI [intrauterine insemination] treatments (one was stopped before insemination) and one private IUI treatment. Also one private failed IVF (treatment stopped before egg collection) and one donor egg IVF. I simply want to be able to create a happy family and bring a new life or lives into the world, to share the joys of sharing with a new human being the wonders of the world.

Before and during my treatments, I have felt hope and optimism. When treatment has been abandoned, I have felt devastated and puzzled as to what I did wrong. Also I have felt angry questioning as to whether I went to the right place and did everything correctly. Infertility has stopped me pushing forward in my career and changing tracks; it has also distanced me from my friends who all have children.

The chances of achieving a pregnancy are dependent upon many factors, such as the quality and quantity of available embryos, the reasons why natural conception is not happening, the history of earlier pregnancies and, most significantly, the age of the potential mother.

Psychological pressures

Janet is 42. She feels that until infertility is recognised as an illness and accepted properly, people will have to pay for private treatment to get what they so desire. It is a silent illness, invisible; no one can tell by looking at you that you are suffering from it.

Janet
We had five treatments in all, paying for two and having three on the NHS. Because of our ages, we paid for the first cycle to get into the process and save time. We acquired money from various sources and went into debt. Not everyone can afford to pay and they just have to wait. Basically, I don't produce enough eggs – I ovulate and have periods but the eggs don't fertilise and both of my tubes are also slightly damaged. Before I was 40, the Ethical Committee was set up and under the guidelines 40 was a cut-off point. Given the choice, I would've carried on but I'd have had a rest for six to twelve months. At the time I was so tired and exhausted, so upset because my body never felt like my own.

I always believed I was put on earth to be a housewife and mother. It is soul-destroying, but my husband is 100 per cent supportive in terms of time and money. We've both been married before – he knew from the start that I couldn't have children, but he stayed with me.

Since undergoing IVF I've had a lot of trouble with depression and am undergoing counselling as I'm not handling the situation well by myself. It helps. I was falling apart, but instead of doing it privately inside I do it openly. Our last go was the best IVF I did as I produced two eggs – my body, however, didn't accept being pregnant. Not to be able to try again was devastating. We could have gone privately, but couldn't afford it. I know I have the steam to go again, but unless you can pay a fortune no one will take you on.

I can't come to terms with being childless; that's why I need counselling and tablets. My husband, Dave, accepts it more than I do. We don't talk about it much now. It's different for a man. I've failed; I'm not complete as a woman because I can't give him a child. He says we're strong enough to cope, but there's a hole there. The treatment becomes part of your life; you don't book holidays – the possibility of becoming parents takes over your life and then it's taken away.

I've never met anyone else with fertility problems – we've never hidden our problems, because we've had support from friends and family. It has affected our relationship, which is very strained. I can't cope; I've changed as a person. It's pulled us apart. My dreams were brushed away over two years ago now – I don't know how I see the future. I think we'll survive. We keep promising ourselves that we'll do things, but he works shifts and we are limited in what we can do as a couple; meanwhile, we are still going through a grieving process. When you see those follicles, they are a person – and then you've lost them. I'd compare it to miscarriage. When the treatment is going on, you are doing something – the buzz is there – now it's like my motor has been switched off.

Dave and I have been very fortunate – we've been involved with all our friends' children. It's helped us enormously to get through it. You can't grieve if children are around: they are a tonic. When my friend told me she was expecting, I was upset but glad. My sister also has two boys. I was so strong when she told me, but sobbed my heart out when she'd gone. She was excited and I couldn't spoil her moment.

We were accepted for adoption and the first application is valid for two years. For a new baby, we need to be 30 or 35 maximum. We could have a teenager or a child with problems. We want a preschool child. I couldn't lose out on that too – I want to bake buns and be a mum. We don't feel strong enough to cope with a badly handicapped child. I couldn't foster – you never know how long you have the children for. Only a baby makes it right.

After the treatment failed I took to comfort eating, but now I have lost 4 stone [25 kilos] so I have achieved something.

I needed Dave very much to hug me, to tell me not to worry. He used to tell me he'd do the worrying. I think that in some ways it made us closer.

I felt strangely proud of myself when I admitted I had a problem and needed serious professional help. My GP arranged for me to see a counsellor, a psychological stress counsellor – it wasn't very helpful. Then she arranged for us to go back to the hospital where we had our IVF and I saw a social worker. On the first visit, I sobbed my heart out because we couldn't have a family. Don't be frightened if you think you need help – go for it sooner rather than later: it gets worse. I hope I'm near the end of my counselling, but I need to know that I can go if I want to. I'm pleased when I take positive steps to change my life and cancel out problems, pleased that I feel more positive and am moving forward.

IVF is not an easy road – it can destroy you and your marriage. A lot of people find it embarrassing to talk about and are frightened to feel upset and want to cry, etc. It is time to speak up to make others aware of the problems. Until infertility is seen as an illness, it won't be treated properly or fairly. Someone at work asked if I had children. I said, 'No, but not through choice.' The conversation ended. It's a little secret world and some treat it like a secret life. Some women have gone through the entire treatment alone (other than the contribution of the sperm in the bottle which she's taken). It is a taboo subject.

Janet has clearly found counselling extremely useful. All of the Assisted Conception Units to whom we spoke for the purposes of researching this book now have counselling available for IVF patients. Counselling is a confidential and sensitive relationship, where the counsellor meets with individuals and couples to discuss the personal, psychological or social effects of their treatment, and its related trauma.

It has long since been recognised that fertility treatment can cause a great deal of stress and anxiety, which often affects both partners and can impact on the ability to cope with domestic, social and working life. People often feel a range of confusing or unusual emotions – depression, anxiety, anger or hostility, guilt, tears, feelings of grief and loss, problems with sleeping or eating and difficulties in coping in social and work situations which would not otherwise be a problem. No one disputes the potential role that emotional disturbance may play in causing infertility problems, although it is hard to prove that psychological trauma is ever the sole cause. Certainly it is true that the hypothalamus (lower brain), which is the major force behind the female reproductive system, is sensitive to psychological stress. In addition, certain drugs, especially tranquillisers and mood-modifiers, can upset the hormonal balance and can temporarily prevent ovulation.

If emotional trauma can create infertility disorders, then there is also no doubt that infertility problems can create emotional trauma, and a self-perpetuating cycle can be formed. Counselling or therapy may help the patients to relax and deal with their stress levels.

Like Janet, Gill wrote that she had never wanted anything in life other than to be a wife and mother. Her letter is full of pain and trauma; she has suffered far more in life than most of us would consider endurable. The following extracts show some of the unnecessary suffering brought on by thoughtlessness and insensitivity.

Gill met Barry while they were both working at a private school.

Gill

Our wedding date was set for mid-July. Barry was six years younger than me, but as I was 27 we decided to start trying for a family before the wedding date. One of my closest friends got married two months after us and she did the same thing, only she became pregnant straight away. I tried not to be envious. As she blossomed my hurt and frustration grew, and there were tears every month when the dreaded period arrived – to say nothing of the small fortune I was spending on pregnancy testing kits.

My wonderfully supportive GP gave me a temperature recording chart and explained that I was most likely to conceive when my temperature changed. He also advised me that it would help if after intercourse I laid with a pillow under my bottom and my feet on the headboard for 30 minutes in order to ensure the maximum amount of seminal fluid was kept inside. Suddenly making love was no longer a spontaneous and beautiful act, but a necessary performance in order to procreate. Barry became understandably resentful of this forced intercourse and the more he complained the more unhappy and unreasonable I became.

At this stage, Gill admitted that her life was far from untroubled. At 19, her first fiancé had committed suicide and in her despair she had turned to drink and finally taken an overdose of drugs. She found that the stress caused by her unsuccessful attempts at conception drove her back to alcohol for solace.

When three months later we still had not conceived, we returned to the doctor. Barry underwent a sperm test which showed an excellent 96 per cent motility – the problem is definitely mine. On reflection, it would have been easier if the problem was shared: I think I could have coped with that better. Now I felt completely to blame – not a real woman and certainly not a proper wife.

I was referred to a gynaecologist. A laparoscopy showed that both of my fallopian tubes were totally blocked and I would need extensive surgery to attempt to rectify the problem. The list for surgery was about 18 months long on the NHS. (I had the laparoscopy privately and was treated like a jewel.)

The operation was carried out on the day after my 29th birthday. I was not at all worried, just excited. After all, my ambition would soon be fulfilled; I would be a mummy. This was just a minor hurdle. How wrong can a person be?

The evening before the operation brought a visit from the physiotherapist, who began to explain aspects of the surgery; then her bleeper went off, so she left me a leaflet and asked me to read it thoroughly. It was written for hysterectomy patients, but I read it from cover to cover. A section explained the importance of sexual abstinence for six weeks after surgery, but I couldn't see that sex was going to be high on my list of priorities straight away.

After the operation I was in agony and I was hugely swollen. The consultant told me that both tubes were completely blocked due to an infection called chlamydia caught some years ago – it is most commonly sexually transmitted. The victim of this infection can be completely unaware of it, but the damage it can do to the female reproductive system can be phenomenal.

In my early 20s I was raped by a taxi driver in Lanzarote, and I had never told Barry about this. There was no way of knowing whether or not this was where I caught the infection, but I found some consolation in believing it to be the case. Fortunately Barry was wonderful and didn't ask for details, so I didn't have to go over the sordid affair with him.

I was ill for six long months after the operation, with recurring infections. After six weeks I went for a post-operative check and was seen by a locum gynaecologist who was lovely. He asked if intercourse was comfortable for us, and we explained that we had followed the guidelines and abstained. He was appalled and explained that damaged fallopian tubes 'fur' up again very quickly after surgery and so we should actually have been as sexually active as possible. Now, six weeks down the line, there was very little chance of my tubes being clear. Sure enough, a dye test showed that my tubes were completely blocked again.

Our next option was IVF, but while we waited we decided to look into adoption – only to discover that you are not permitted to be on an adoption list if you are undergoing or awaiting IVF treatment. The age limit for baby adoption in Cumbria at this time was 34, and the wait for a baby on average was three to four years. So we lied and said that we had declined IVF – close family and good friends also had to lie for us. The adoption procedure is very stringent, and we struggled through group meetings, interviews, police checks, financial checks and so on. Finally, we fell down on the medicals – my GP assured me that he did not need to mention my attempted suicide since it was so long ago, but then he accidentally included it in his report and the social workers explained that, since I had tried to cover this up, I may have hidden other things too and we were thus unfit to have a normal baby. We were told that we could, however, be offered a physically or mentally handicapped child, which made me absolutely furious: if we were unfit to have a normal child, how could we be good enough for a disabled child? These special children take so much more looking after. Are all of these poor kiddies placed with second-rate citizens?

Our marriage got into big difficulties. Barry really didn't know how to cope with my distress; I think being six years younger didn't help. I was unnecessarily hard on him and he began to stay out late with his single mates. My drinking accelerated.

At last we had an appointment at the IVF clinic at Newcastle. I had to take a nasal spray four times each day and Perganol injected intramuscularly each morning. I felt terrible and looked awful, and then our first course had to stop as my blood pressure went sky high. We went back on to the waiting list. Our marriage went from bad to worse, Barry was never in, and when he was we argued. He began lashing out and I got drunk. I met Tommy, a widower who is 18 years my senior. I found I could talk to him and he really understood. The inevitable happened and we started to have an affair.

In the meantime our second IVF attempt came up and this time all went well, with nine good eggs ready for collection. I went in for a preliminary scan, only to find that all the eggs had died – something inside me had killed them. I cannot begin to describe the torment. Barry and I took a holiday in Spain, which was disastrous. I knew now that I was in love with Tommy. Barry and I were tearing each other apart, and in the end it just happened I left and never went back. I moved in with Tommy and his adult sons, and three weeks later another girl moved in with Barry.

After that, Gill suffered what she saw as dreadful prejudice, particularly from the wife of one of Tommy's sons, who conceived and delivered a baby girl, Tommy's first grandchild. The mother would not allow the baby in the house with Gill, nor would she accept gifts or cards from her, accusing Gill of an unhealthy interest in other people's babies. Gill wrote, in conclusion:

I definitely feel that as an infertile person you are often treated as a second-class citizen, an outcast. People either rattle on endlessly about their own kids, assuming it will make you feel better. Or there is the 'you don't know how lucky you are' brigade, saying 'I'd give my right arm to be in your shoes, you should have my kids for a weekend, you be glad you are as you are.' Alternatively people simply clam up and avoid you.

Babies are a fact of life – it's been pointed out to me often enough. That doesn't alter the fact that having a baby is the most natural thing in the world. Even insects can manage it – so why can't I?

I watched a chat show on infertility once. A 74-year-old woman phoned up. She had experienced most forms of grief in her life, and in time all the pain got easier except for the pain of infertility. I sympathise with her. If anything, I find it getting harder as I get older and time for the magic cure runs out. I know the pain will never leave me, awake or asleep. Some days are good, others are bad.

IUI (interuterine insemination)

IUI involves the intramuscular or subcutaneous injections of human menopausal gonadatrophins. Vaginal ultrasound scans are then used to assess follicle growth. When the desired growth is achieved, an injection of human chorionic gonadatrophin (HCG) is given to induce ovulation – this takes place usually 34 to 38 hours after the HCG injection. About two hours before insemination, the male provides a fresh semen sample, which is prepared with 'sperm wash' techniques. This involves diluting the sperm sample with culture medium in a test tube, centrifuging the mixture and leaving a sperm pellet which is then suspended in fresh culture medium, allowing the sperm to swim up into the top layer of the medium. It sounds technical, but the object is to isolate the best quality sperm to be harvested for insemination. The insemination itself is performed using a fine catheter to deposit the sperm into the uterine cavity via the cervix, a process which can be performed on an out-patient basis.

Like GIFT, IUI is used for cases of unexplained infertility, cervical mucus hostility and mild male factor problems such as low sperm motility. It has the advantage of being less invasive than other methods, and can be performed in centres with limited resources. The success rate, however, is only 10–20 per cent and there is again a risk of multiple birth.

Caroline, our next contributor, is able to offer her own experiences of the comparison between IUI and IVF.

Caroline
After six months of trying to conceive we saw the doctor and were referred to the hospital where I had various blood tests which confirmed I was ovulating. My husband went for sperm tests which confirmed he had a slightly low count, but there was nothing to worry about. We went away and kept on trying. After a year we went back to our doctor and asked to be referred to a private hospital (covered under insurance) for further tests. Yes, I was ovulating but there was a problem with the sperm. I actually got to look at the sperm under the microscope, which was fascinating, if disappointing, as most of the sperm were inactive or abnormal. The sperm did not have a very long lifespan and although my husband had a normal sperm count, most of the sperm were abnormal, a fact not picked up by the NHS hospital earlier.

The next stage was for me to undergo a laparoscopy operation, which consists of two incisions to the stomach, enabling the doctor to pass dye through the tubes to check they are clear. I was scared, as I'd never had an operation before. I came out of the anaesthetic very well, but sore, as if a horse had kicked me in the stomach – very tender. The doctor came round to see us in the evening – I had endometriosis, which I had never heard of. One of my tubes was plastered to the back of my pelvis and I had a cyst which they managed to remove. Our chances of conceiving normally were less than 1 per cent. IVF was the only realistic option.

I lay in bed thinking they must have got this wrong. I am the healthiest person, my periods are as regular as clockwork – although heavy and painful. I thought this showed how fertile I was. WRONG! When the doctor left the room we both cried uncontrollably and that was the beginning of our emotional roller-coaster. Why us? We had everything to offer a baby.

IVF was going to cost us £2,000, so I looked into the NHS to see what our chances of treatment were. We were not entitled to IVF treatment on the NHS as my tubes were not completely blocked and also my husband had a high abnormal sperm count. The only people entitled were women who had completely blocked tubes and men who had completely normal sperm – both under 35 years of age. I wrote to the NHS to complain about entitlement to IVF and was told that only a limited amount of funding was put aside each year, so there had to be strict criteria regarding entitlement. I also wrote to my MP to complain and am still waiting for an answer eight months on. We went privately.

My first understanding of IVF was a glossy book idea of a test tube baby. How romantic. How wonderful. How WRONG. Nothing could prepare us for such an emotional nightmare.

Treatment started with injections to the stomach – not good with my phobia about needles. I couldn't even look at a needle, let alone inject myself. I had already fainted giving blood samples, but my husband was taught how to administer the injection and I just lay back and thought of babies. What a terrific husband and what guts. He knew he had to be quick, so wham bam he injected me and we left with our bag of needles and drugs. After about a week I had to start on my second injection. My stomach was beginning to go blue and yellow, but I was almost word perfect on singing songs from *The*

Sound of Music while being injected. I developed an allergic
reaction to the second drug, so that was even more painful. After
a month I was feeling very battered and very emotional.

I had been back and forth to the hospital for scans to see how
many eggs I was producing and I had a total of 13 follicles so
I was now ready for egg collection. My last injection was at
midnight before egg collection the next day – the glass drug
capsule shattered in my hand and we had to scoop up what we
could, avoiding the glass. Egg collection was a simple procedure,
I thought – under anaesthetic – but I was wheeled back to my
room in extreme pain: no one told me how much it would hurt.
The final indignity was an injection to my bottom to maintain
my womb lining.

On leaving hospital all I could do was cry. I began to have
bladder trouble; I could hardly walk, so the doctor came out to
visit and within the hour an ambulance came to take me to A
& E. My bladder had gone into retention. A catheter was fitted
and I was given drugs. They wanted to keep me in, but my eggs
were being replaced the following day so I had to leave. We rang
the private hospital the next day to be told only six eggs had
fertilised. Another girl came in who had her eggs collected on
the same day – she was bounding down the corridor and my
husband and I looked at each other in disbelief at how two
people could react so differently.

Insemination went according to plan, without any hitches,
and we were told to come back in two weeks for a pregnancy
test. We asked for the other three eggs to be frozen but were told
they were not good enough. We went away and continued with
the injections to maintain my womb lining. The pregnancy test
was returned negative. One word and it was as if my heart had
stopped. I sat in a state of utter shock and disbelief. My husband
sat and just cried. I maintained my composure until we got to
the car, then cried uncontrollably. We had been through so
much. We were both gutted, exhausted and needed to go away
and lick our wounds. On arrival home there was a letter from
a friend I hadn't seen for a while, saying, 'Guess what, terrific
news, I'm pregnant.'

Six months later we received a note from the NHS hospital
saying I could start IUI treatment. We were excited and eager,
as IUI is a lot less intense and I was relieved not to have to go
through the jabs and egg collection. It sounded very attractive
despite only a 10 per cent success rate per treatment. I got a
prescription from my doctor for my drugs, only to find there

is a national shortage and the drugs company that has 85 per cent of the market is having problems.

We started injections on the first day of my period – one injection every other day into my bottom (least painful). A week later I had to attend hospital for a scan to see whether I had an 18 mm egg – I did, which meant insemination in three days. I returned equipped with my pot of fresh sperm keeping warm under my armpit. Waiting to be inseminated was a bit like a cattle market – us all queuing up like a load of heifers. Insemination was straightforward; I was left to lie on my back for ten minutes and then left. It was 99 per cent less stressful than IVF, and 99 per cent less emotional; exciting even, thoroughly recommended and you do not put all your hopes in one go at it.

Our first attempt was unsuccessful, but we are trying IUI until we have enough money saved for more IVF.

My infertility is a taboo subject which friends don't know how to tackle – or don't want to. At first my husband didn't want to tell anyone about our infertility. He bottled it all up and was beginning to make himself ill. I preferred to offload this big burden and assured my husband that if people know they can help and support you. People have reacted in two ways. My closest friends have been an absolute nightmare and have alienated us from our circle as they find the situation just too embarrassing. Family, work and my husband's friends have been wonderful and fully supportive throughout. I think it is at a time like this when you need people to support you, but must not be too disappointed if others don't fully understand. People follow our progress with interest now and we discuss our infertility openly. I feel that if any of our friends should find themselves in a similar situation, I want them to know that it is not something to be swept under the carpet – people are leaving having a family till later in life now and are finding complications which are becoming all too common. I don't want them to suffer in silence like we first did – it's OK to admit to infertility because it can be treated.

Costs and related difficulties

Critical questions, which all couples contemplating the trauma of infertility treatment must ask themselves, are how many cycles are needed, on average, to achieve pregnancy, and at what point to stop trying. Each treatment cycle is a 'new ball game', and the odds of pregnancy (and this is pregnancy, not live birth, for which the odds are even lower) are about 20 per cent each time. If the pregnancy 'takes', but miscarries some time later, the couple must decide all over again whether they want to try the in vitro procedure again.

These are clearly emotionally loaded questions, and the decision about when to give up depends largely on the feelings of the couple involved.

IVF can be extremely expensive, since most couples have to take time away from work, travel long distances, and often pay for hotel accommodation for two weeks or longer during each attempted cycle.

Moira's account, which follows, is particularly relevant, since it outlines the direct costs of fertility treatment in 1995.

Moira

I got married some years ago to a divorced man, the father of two children. When we were first together I was on the pill and then when we decided to have children I came off the pill and nothing happened. As my husband was 26 years older than me his opinion was that if it happened it happened and if it didn't it didn't. Through the next 15 years nothing ever happened and as we were living in Spain I never sought out any help. Sadly after a few years my husband died.

I then met another man whom I married. Peter is a kind, loving, caring friend, husband and lover. When I had not fallen pregnant after six months I sought assistance from our local GP. I told him my story and he agreed to start tests. I had monthly blood tests for three months and Peter had semen analysis tests. I was then put on Clomid for six months. Still nothing happened. An appointment was made for me to have a laparoscopy and dye to check out my tubes and womb for blockages, etc. This proved to be satisfactory, but they found a lump the size of a grapefruit. I was admitted to hospital within a week for the lump to be removed. They diagnosed endometriosis and removed the lump and also one of my ovaries. When I got over this operation they told me they thought the only way I would get pregnant would be by IVF.

Again I went back to my GP who, although sympathetic, told me IVF could not be funded by the health authority and that we would have to pay ourselves. Norfolk and Norwich do not fund anything, not even the drugs. However, he did recommend that we visit Bourn Hall at Cambridge.

I got the Bourn Hall brochure and worked out the prices which we could afford and after long talks decided we would try it. We estimated it would cost around £3,500 for the first attempt.

In March we had the initial consultation and were shown around and everything was discussed as to what we would be up against. I was examined and Peter had to have a semen analysis test. We were accepted as potential IVF candidates pending blood tests for HIV, hepatitis and some other blood tests for me. Bourn explained they could do the tests, which again would cost us, or we could get our local GP to do them.

INITIAL CONSULTATION £120
SEMEN ANALYSIS £45

We came home and made an appointment with our GP to ask for blood tests. We were refused because they were for infertility and we are not funded for infertility. We were really annoyed, because if I'd gone in and lied and said I had slept with someone else they would have done an HIV test as routine. My GP agreed and said to leave it to him. Two days later he rang and told me they had had a group practice meeting and had agreed on this occasion to do our blood tests. Made me feel like they were doing me a big favour.

The blood test results were all clear and treatment was ready to begin on day two of my next period.

In May I got my period and rang Bourn Hall. I arranged for a scan and blood tests. At Bourn Hall I was given the prescription for my drugs and the nurse showed me how to inject myself.

DRUGS £1,129

Following blood tests I discovered that I couldn't start the treatment as my FSH blood level was too high.

CHARGE FOR TESTS £175

In June we went through the same routine. Problem with the scan this time. No go.

CHARGE FOR TESTS £100

By July we felt a bit despondent. Blood and scan again.

CHARGE FOR IVF £2,490

I rang at 3 o'clock. Yes, yes, yes. I was so excited I cried. I cleared the dressing table in the spare room – it looked more like an operating theatre with all the drugs and syringes. I wasn't at all nervous, just happy.

The following day I had a scan and blood tests. It was deemed necessary to increase the dosage of Metrodin but I didn't care. It was still another hurdle nearer.

I needed to get more drugs because of the higher dosage.

MORE DRUGS £46

In July I had a scan and blood tests and had to see my doctor. Apparently I wasn't responding to treatment. The doctor advised us to abandon the treatment and opt instead to use a donor egg. I felt gutted. We were entitled to a refund on the £2,490. We were only charged for the three visits.

CHARGE FOR VISITS £575

It had seemed such a waste of time and money when nothing has come out of it. We are still discussing donor eggs. There is also a waiting list of 15 months and the cost they tell us is £4,500 plus drugs, so once again another £6,000 approximately.

Not everyone is successful and it certainly costs more than anticipated. We don't know yet what we will do. It is still early days, as it was only yesterday that I became a total failure.

Angela, who closes this chapter for us, gives us an insider's view of the importance of the medical team involved in the fertility treatment. Angela has happily put herself into the hands of one particular clinic four times and trusts its staff implicitly – this trust is vital to her psychological outlook in her continued aspirations.

Angela
I am 31 years old, married with one son who will be eleven in December 1996. His name is Ashley and he was born when I

was 20; we have been trying for almost ten years for a brother or sister for him. I have had all the tests going, and I also had tubal surgery when I was about 25. Six months later when nothing was happening I started on IVF. At the time I would have done anything to have a child and I'm sure would have hurt anyone who got in my way. We visited Bourn Hall and after talking things over decided to wait a while. I went back to work full-time and tried to get my life into some sort of order.

During the years of waiting our life was happy although Graham knew that I would have given anything to have had a baby. Then in February 1995 we met Professor [Lord Robert] Winston. He seemed to me the only person in the world who really understood how I felt and it was then I knew that the Hammersmith in London was the place where I felt happy to be treated; we booked for March/April of that year. I can remember each step of the treatment, it was so exciting. Even the injections and the sore bum were wonderful because the prospects looked good. I had two good embryos implanted and waited the longest two weeks of my life. Nothing can prepare you for this kind of waiting. I did everything right – I rested and even took time off work. Still the result was negative. To say I was brokenhearted was the understatement of the year. I couldn't believe that life could be so cruel. I felt I had nothing left to live for, but life has to go on.

We booked again for August/September. Just the same. Sailed through the treatments with the help of a very good friend, Michelle, who was then attempting her fourth IVF. We had two good embryos replaced, although this time we had asked for three, but once again – nothing. I felt very empty and disappointed again, but was determined to find the money for another try. Can you believe it! All those injections and sniffing again.

The third time was not so easy as I felt sick all the time and was very tearful. However, I managed with the support of my good friends and the Hammersmith team. Egg collection and embryo transfer time again and this time we did persuade the doctors to implant three, but still nothing. Another bitter disappointment and even Graham this time could not comfort me. Why me? Why is life so cruel? Friends and family told me I should be grateful that I had one child, but nothing took away the longing and the hurt.

This brings us nearly up to date. I started my fourth attempt in June and it has been wonderful. My doctor has been so very good to me with my drugs and he is 100 per cent supportive. The staff at the Hammersmith too have been wonderful. We had 13 eggs collected; nine of them fertilised and three very special ones were implanted. Another agonising wait for results – and another bitter, bitter disappointment.

Five days later and I'm determined to raise another £1,600 for my fifth, and final, attempt. We were treated so well by the unit that we donated our spare embryos to research into repeated IVF failures being carried out by two doctors at the Hammersmith.

Our family now tells us to give it up as a bad job, but we feel we've been through so much together that we can't give up yet. IVF is a very important part of our lives now, and although we may not have had the result we long for at least it is giving us hope.

We are so grateful to all the people who have helped us so very much – Professor Winston and all the Hammersmith team, Michelle, Glyn and Cen and everyone else who put up with looking at my backside for three to four weeks at each attempt.

If I were to give advice to a first-timer it would be to get your home and life in order first. I read somewhere, 'Put IVF into your life. Not your life into IVF.' Easier said than done.

The treatment is painful, very tiring and very expensive. We have spent £6,000 so far in only just over a year with more to go. Get good friends and family behind you. You will need them.

IVF is my only chance to have another child. I don't know what my future holds. But I've got ten embryo pictures framed and put safely away. They are my babies. They're not here, but I loved them and cried for each and every one of them.

6 Alternative decisions on treatment

Once a couple have come to terms with their infertility issues, a range of opportunities are open to them. In this chapter we attempt to cover some of the alternatives.

Catherine opens with her well-formed views on fertility treatment, and their overall impact on a person's life.

Catherine

I attempted an IVF treatment but only developed three follicles, which the doctors felt was not enough to do an IVF on. This was in spite of the fact that I was taking six ampoules of oestrogen daily, so instead I had another IUI, which went very well, and I continued to take the injections to the end of the cycle. An American counsellor friend of mine sent me an especially made positive visualisation tape, which I listened to every day of the treatment. It was called 'Catherine's Meadow' and full of wonderful images of walking through fields and woods and by the sea. It helped to relax me and made me hopeful and excited.

I kept as positive as I was able, and when the treatment hadn't worked in the end it really was hell. Over the next few days, I felt positively wrung out and twisted with grief and pain. We went away for a few days and went to a wonderful ancient woodland looking for mushrooms. It was drizzling heavily and I became blinded with tears, not seeing anything. I felt so awful, I wanted to die. With the pouring rain, the falling leaves and my tears, I wanted just to lie down and cry and cry. I thought I'd be crying forever.

Two months later we had a consultation with a doctor in a recommended hospital in London, as we decided that if we were going to give IVF another chance we should go for the best available. The consultant there told me that because of my age (39) there was only a 10–15 per cent chance of success. This was very disappointing as I had understood that the success rate would be 30 per cent. However, we made a provisional arrangement to go ahead. After a holiday we were able to get a better perspective on things and decided not to go any further with the IVF programme.

This is chiefly because we have both been getting more interested in health, nutrition and the organic movement. Somehow, it seems the very antithesis of the invasive technology of IVF and all its side effects. Then there's the trauma and the cost. We joined the preconceptual care organisation Foresight. One of their aims is to achieve an optimum state of nutritional health. Following a hair analysis, we are now on a four-month programme of vitamins and minerals and we are eating healthy foods. This way we feel more in control of our lives. It was not an easy decision to make to let the option of IVF go, in the face of all the publicity and media attention on IVF. One somehow feels it should be pursued regardless, because it's there. We may reconsider it, although I'm aware that my fertility is now supposed to plummet when I reach 40.

I am now seeing a counsellor every month but deep down there is still the pain. However, I do not want to spend the next five years distraught over it all and am looking at ways of making my life more meaningful and creative. It is sometimes horrendous to realise that over all these years, I had the assumption that I would be a mother. I truly feel like a tree that is stuck, prevented from growing branches and flowers and expanding. It is both a physical and mental pain/frustration. I don't want to be so miserable. I am subject to feeling such negativity and hopelessness and a sense of gloom and failure at times. It really permeates everything.

Much of this book has dwelt on those who opt for infertility treatment. Like Catherine, Barbara reminds us that it is equally proactive to decide against such invasive processes.

Barbara

My husband and I stopped using contraception to start a family. After ten months I fell pregnant, but at eleven weeks I had mild stomach pains and some bleeding. The pregnancy ended in miscarriage. Meantime, all my female friends and colleagues appeared to be getting pregnant, and a year later I visited the doctor as I felt I should be pregnant by then. His referral to the infertility clinic showed me to be ovulating, but that I had high prolactin levels. The consultant bluntly informed me, following her examination, that I had either polycystic ovaries or possibly a pituitary tumour. Ultrasound three weeks later showed an ovarian cyst. I later had a laparoscopy, which showed clear fallopian tubes but mild to moderate endometriosis – I had never heard of it. I started a six-month course of Danazol. Each time I visited the clinic, I spoke to a different doctor who gave me different stories – some were positive and some negative about my endometriosis preventing pregnancy. Ultrasound showed the cyst had reduced in size.

I again became pregnant (according to a home test) but my period started a week later. In time, I was called to the clinic to attend a post-coital test – I arrived as instructed but they forgot me, so by the time I had the test it was two hours after intercourse and this was very upsetting. The test showed a low number of 'live' sperm, which did not surprise me. They asked me to return another time, but I said, 'No thanks.'

I decided to stop going to the clinic and let nature decide. I am not religious, but do not believe too much in interfering with my body. However, the hardest part of the endometriosis (which is painful) is not that we may not have children, but that it is the social norm to have them. After all, in Italy 62-year-old women have them [see Chapter 7]. I would like to see better trained staff in infertility clinics, but of course the resources are not there. I will not become a woman obsessed with wanting her own children or resentful of others, as luckily I have many nieces and nephews nearby and they do remind us of how much work they entail.

The following letter tells not just of failure in fertility treatment, but of the failure of the health service to monitor and counsel a patient.

Joan

In June, having not conceived for a couple of years, we went to see a GP who advised us to have some tests with a consultant. The waiting list was six months plus, and the GP suggested we went privately.

We saw a consultant and had the relevant tests. He said my eggs were not mature enough and he would give me two months' supply of Clomid. He said one in 25 on the drug conceived twins. He mentioned no side effects.

I waited for my period and to our surprise we had a positive pregnancy result. I rang the consultant's secretary to cancel my next appointment as it was no longer necessary. I received a letter from the consultant saying, 'Congratulations. See you in my antenatal clinic.'

I rang my GP. (We were now referred back to the NHS.) I saw him and asked if it was possible to have an early scan because I had been on fertility drugs. He said no. He did not examine me. He said to make an appointment in a few weeks with the midwife.

I was ten weeks pregnant, and saw a midwife. I was feeling very large and bloated. I mentioned this to her. She did not examine me but said most people on Clomid only have one baby.

I rang the midwife for my scan date – not till 18 weeks. I complained of feeling big and sore down below. She said it was normal, and that my dates were probably wrong. This is not possible on Clomid.

At 14 weeks I spoke to the midwife. I told her that I could feel kicking, but she replied 'It's only wind.' She told me to come in for some tests. I did, and saw the midwife, who listened to the heartbeat. She didn't try both sides to maybe pick up two heartbeats.

By 16 weeks I was feeling very big and my vagina was swollen. I went to see if I could see a midwife, but instead I saw a lady doctor. She said my dates must be wrong.

At 18 weeks I had a scan. I could see two babies on screen. I started to feel elated when suddenly I was told, 'You have four babies.' The shock was traumatic and devastating. I already had a 4-year-old. How was I going to cope with four babies? All I could think about was my little boy and how were we going to cope.

I saw the consultant, who was shell-shocked to say the least. He said to come in for a cervical stitch to keep the babies in. He told me to take vitamin C and that I would have to come into hospital at 26 weeks for bed rest. I would deliver at 36 weeks.

The consultant informed surgery that day that I was expecting quads. I was given the number of a Twin Support Club in

Exeter. Then I spoke to Social Services to see what benefits might be available, but found there was no help going. I was told to ring the health visitor. I spoke to Tamba [Twins and Multiple Birth Association] – but there was no help available there either. Super Twins Plus sent me a list of secondhand pushchairs, etc.

My GP never rang or visited. A friend asked my midwife if she would call as I was distressed. I rang the health visitor. No one came. Eventually I did see the midwife. She gave me no advice, just saying, 'It's amazing what you can do.'

Everything was going round in my head – cots, prams, etc. How would I ever go out, feeding four babies? I really thought I would be bringing four babies home. I even bought four premature baby-gros as I knew they would be small. I was very tearful, confused and frightened. Not one person came round to talk to me apart from a midwife when a friend told her I was desperate.

I was beginning to wish I had never taken the drugs. Tried to carry on as normal. It was Christmas and I didn't want it to affect our little boy.

The Wednesday after Christmas I was due to go in for my cervical stitch. My husband spoke to his brother, a GP. He couldn't understand why I hadn't been scanned. Most fertility patients are scanned earlier. I overheard him mention that the babies might be handicapped, and I broke down in tears. I said I didn't want them inside me any more. The question of termination arose.

I saw the consultant. He said we could have a selective termination at ten to twelve weeks, but it was clearly too late for that. The chances of having all four babies alive and well were not good.

I had a termination of the pregnancy. I did not see the babies. I gave birth with sheets over my head: I was very frightened to see them. I had to go into theatre for removal of the placentas. I went home next day, and the midwife came round for a few days.

To this day my GP has never made contact. I changed doctor.

We had a funeral and buried our babies.

After such a traumatic time I struggle each day to come to terms with what happened. The guilt is unbearable. I never stop thinking about what I have done. Nobody knows I terminated my babies apart from family. I feel as if I'm living a lie. I wonder if they would have survived or not. The only thing I have of them is a photo in my lounge. They are part of my family and always will be. The regrets of not seeing them and not holding them are there and the regrets of terminating them are also there. Part of me has died inside, feeling so lost and empty and very let down by the medical profession.

I received counselling, which helped for a while.

I also had an apology from the consultant. He gave me Clomid again – a lower dosage – and I was scanned every month.

Nine months went by and I was still not pregnant. The feelings left after the termination were devastating. I felt I was being punished for terminating my babies. I wanted them and I loved them.

Eventually I came off fertility treatment.

It has all been emotionally draining and I am still trying to cope with my loss. I have very mixed emotions.

Finally my period was late. I took a test and was thrilled with a positive result. It seemed a miracle as I am not on any drugs. Sadly I miscarried ten days later.

After waiting eleven months, I had a laparoscopy test to see if there was any tubal damage.

I am now awaiting an appointment to see the consultant.

GIFT (gamete intrafallopian transfer)

GIFT is considered by some to be the cheaper, less sophisticated version of IVF; it usually offers shorter queues, and doesn't require the sophisticated equipment needed by IVF for embryo culture. The cost per treatment is around £1,200 if a GP covers the cost of the necessary drugs.

The GIFT procedure involves daily Buserilin injections into the abdomen to suppress the natural hormone cycle, followed by Perganol, a hormone stimulant, then an ultrasound scan to assess the development of the eggs. If good-quality eggs develop, they are collected under a general anaesthetic using a laparoscopy (this is also needed to guide the surgeon when replacing the eggs and sperm in the fallopian tubes). Unfortunately there is no confirmation that fertilisation has taken place (unlike IVF, where fertilisation occurs in the petri dish), and there is a danger of hyper-stimulation syndrome where excessive fluid leaks from blood vessels into body cavities – a potentially fatal condition. GIFT can, however, be a useful technique for couples with unexplained infertility.

For GIFT to work, the woman needs to have patent (clear) fallopian tubes. It can be helpful where the woman has cervical mucus hostility or where there are mild male factor problems such as low sperm motility. One advantage is that fertilisation occurs in the natural environment – the fallopian tube – but there are risks attached, particularly the need for general anaesthetic and the risk of multiple birth (if two or three eggs are fertilised). It can also be seen as a disadvantage that the couple involved do not know whether or not fertilisation has taken place – they have to wait and see what happens.

Sue wrote to us with a delightful account of her experience of GIFT and very thoughtfully asked her husband, Miller, to provide his own views. Since it is rare to hear from the men involved in fertility treatment, we offer their story from his side of the picture. Incidentally, it is of interest to note that their child was the last to be born to their fertility clinic through GIFT – it has now been completely superseded by IVF.

Sue and Miller

I got married at 24 to Sue, a woman one year older than myself, after living together for about a year. We were happy and confident that we had made the right choice in partners. Sue came off the pill just before we got married and we intended to have children as soon as they came along. Nothing planned or rushed, but let nature take its course and bless us when things were right.

A year passed with no sign of children. I was not concerned myself, and was enjoying discovering my marriage and the pleasures of married life without the responsibilities of children. Sue, on the other hand, was becoming concerned and asked if I minded her visiting the doctor. I didn't mind and even agreed to accompany her. We were laughed out of the surgery. That description may be a little harsh, as we were simply advised that it was far too early to be worrying and we should go away and relax and let nature take its course. We followed this advice and left it for another year, but all this time Sue was convinced that there was something wrong.

We returned to the doctor a year later and were again given some basic advice and assured that nature would take its course. Another year passed and feeling that there was the possibility that Sue's worry was contributing to the problem the doctor referred us to an infertility clinic. The first step was to ask us to undergo some basic tests. BASIC! The most embarrassing tests you can think of. For myself it went something like this: 'Take this bottle and go home. Do not have any kind of sexual contact for four days and then masturbate into the bottle. Put the bottle into a brown paper bag and return it to the hospital. Take it to a department full of young women and hand it over the counter.' For Sue it was even worse: 'Climb on to this couch and remove your clothes from the waist down. Open your legs while we explore and inflict pain without telling you why.'

We were again told to go home and relax, maybe have a holiday, but don't think about it. Six months later we returned for another go – more tests. This time it involved Sue spending a couple of days in hospital while they put some tubes and a camera inside her to have a look around.

Then the dreaded day arrived when we were asked to return to see our doctor for the test results. More than two years had passed since bringing this to the doctor's attention and nearly four since getting married. Sue was now 30 and I was approaching 29. We sat in the doctor's surgery, holding hands and fearing the worst. The doctor pulled no punches and told us straight. There was a problem, but they were unsure what it was. We were shown a report from the hospital, where it described Sue as a geriatric woman, slightly overweight, married to a young virile man. This was explained as meaning that Sue was getting on for a potential mother, whereas I had another 50 possible years ahead to become a father. The finger was being pointed quite squarely at Sue as the source of the problem. My instant reaction was one of relief, but then within minutes it dawned on me that Sue would be feeling terrible.

We left the surgery confused and deflated. I tried everything to assure Sue that it made no difference to me or my feelings towards her, but nothing seemed to get through. I am sure that Sue saw on my face the relief in the surgery, but I continued to try everything to convince her that we were in this together all the way. Over the next few days I convinced myself that having children would make no difference to me or my relationship with Sue.

Weeks passed as we awaited our next appointment and suddenly Sue came up with a suggestion I will never forget. She felt that she had let me down and would release me from my marriage vows if that was the path I wished to follow. I cried with her for hours, but she was inconsolable. She even suggested that I could have children by another woman if I wanted to. Again and again I tried to explain that Sue giving me children was not the reason for me asking her to marry me.

We suddenly received a letter from the hospital advising us that we were being transferred from the infertility clinic across to the fertility clinic next door. This brought new hope and lifted Sue. We attended our first appointment only to be let down again. We were going to have to repeat all the tests and follow another two-year plan of tests, counselling and consultations. At the end of this time the only option left was fertility treatment.

I was sure that we had to remain a couple through all of this and made sure I never missed an appointment or hospital visit. I would sit in the waiting room among half a dozen women who had attended the clinic on their own. I would continue to supply samples in little bottles hidden inside brown paper bags and delivered red-faced to this room of young gossiping women. I even accompanied Sue when she attended a counselling session with a therapist – a young girl who was supposedly going to get us through the heartache of failure. When she suggested we take up art therapy I could take no more.

We even looked at adoption as an option. Being adopted myself I am very aware that things can go terribly wrong. I feel strongly that adoption should be for the child's sake and not the parents' sake. If you are considering adoption as an option to fill a gap in your life, then prepare for disaster. In our case, Sue was so desperate for a child of her own that no other child would have been enough to fill the gap she felt was there. Thankfully Sue saw my point and we dropped the idea for the time being.

Years passed until one day we were contacted with an offer to join a professor who was performing some GIFT trials. At last we started to see some real action. Suddenly we started to see the consultants and senior registrars. After all this time we had never been asked a very basic, but simple question. Did we actually know how to reproduce? I was still convinced that I was doing all of this for Sue and I would happily walk away from it without regret. We suddenly came across another barrier that could put a stop to the whole thing. Funding. It was explained to us that there was very limited funding for this procedure, and because the success rate was very low we might have to contribute financially if they failed on the first attempt. Sue was at breaking point and there was no discussion needed. We had to continue now whatever the cost. No amount of money, time or effort would be too much now. Sue was desperate to try anything.

We continued until the magic time when our names reached the top of a very long waiting list of other couples – waiting for the same procedure. We had by now been given a new GP within the same health practice and she was totally supportive, even to the point of agreeing to write us a prescription for the drugs needed to proceed. It was on. We entered two different hospitals, Sue to have her part of the operation and myself 7 miles away [11 km] to give yet another sample. Sue had both the eggs and sperm implanted later that afternoon and returned home the following day. Then came the waiting. And waiting and a little more waiting. Although we knew that we had to return to the hospital 14 days later for a pregnancy test, it was killing us. We walked in on that 14th day and sat in the waiting room holding hands and whispering like schoolchildren. We were called in and told the bad news. It had not worked and we needed to start all over again. A minimum of three months needed to pass before we could have another attempt.

We were deflated and silent. There was nothing that needed to be said and nothing worth saying. We would try again and again if need be.

Then one morning, about 18 days later, Sue asked if I thought she should have started her period, or if the process could have messed things up? I could see a sparkle in her eyes and a hopeful smile on her face. We ran to the chemist and bought a home tester kit that confirmed our dreams. Sue was on the phone within seconds and insisted on speaking to the clinic's manager. We were assured that there could not be any mistake and we were grasping at straws, but they agreed to retest that morning. We both sat by the phone and waited and dived for every call coming through. Late in the afternoon they rang and apologised for their mistake. Yes, Sue was pregnant and they would like to see us as soon as possible.

George Edward was born nine months and one week later. I cried and cried. Who had I been trying to fool!? Not bothered if I have children or not? I wanted the whole world to know the joy I felt. Sue was on cloud nine and had got her dream.

Through all of this, something had not occurred to me until it was all over. As the woman in this, with a large family and many friends, Sue had found many people to talk with, cry with and share the heartache and worry. As the man, in a society that still expects us to put on a brave face, I was expected to face this alone. Male friends and family just did not understand or want to know about the details of failure and sorrow. I had lied to myself in an attempt to hide the feelings and inner pain. I had tried to put on this brave face and be the strong one in the relationship, but looking down at the tiny little bundle in my arms I suddenly knew what it was all about.

We left the hospital with our little miracle and a happiness in our hearts that nobody will ever be able to take away.

Alison also experienced the GIFT technique, but is one of the lucky women for whom treatment is, eventually, unnecessary.

Alison
I am 30 years old and have a beautiful daughter after nine years of trying for a baby. I have polycystic ovaries and have been on GIFT as well as tablets and injections.

I started on Clomiphene at 21 years old and thought I would get pregnant on it straight away. Nothing happened, so I was sent for a laparoscopy and then for an internal scan. I was led to believe that my problems would soon be overcome. I was given injections to stimulate my ovaries, laser treatment, another laparoscopy and then the cysts were burned away. Still hopeful.

I went back to the hospital to find that the cysts had already returned. This was a big blow to both of us.

After years of toing and froing with all kinds of treatments, I was told that they couldn't do anything more for me. I was devastated and asked if I could go on IVF treatment. The consultant said that because there was nothing wrong with my tubes I could go on GIFT.

I waited for two years on the NHS waiting list. The waiting procedure is similar to IVF. I had to take Primulet N to make me have a period. I was very moody on this and had many arguments with my husband. I felt like my head was going to explode. I also had a nasal spray which I had to use twice a day, better than Buserilin which I'd had to use three times a day.

I was then started on Metrodin injections, which made me feel great, really well, and my hormones levelled out. Although I kept saying I wasn't setting my heart on getting pregnant, deep down I was looking forward to GIFT because I thought it would be successful.

All the scans were great. I had about ten eggs and my womb thickness was correct. I felt great.

The day came for my GIFT. Everything went well. The doctor came round next day and told me they had put three eggs back. I was over the moon and thought that I was pregnant. After the two weeks I still hadn't had a period so we went for a test at the hospital. The embryologist told us that the eggs had fertilised so we were even more hopeful.

The result came back – negative. We were devastated and both cried. I couldn't speak to anyone. Family and friends were ringing but I would just burst into tears. This was a very hard time for us, especially as I felt I'd let my husband down. Our marriage went through quite a rocky patch. Great strain on a wife, especially if she is working and having to fit in all the treatments, etc.

Eighteen months later I was called to go on the GIFT again. I had a pregnancy test done before I started any treatment. And to everyone's amazement I was seven weeks pregnant. It seems that in forgetting about getting pregnant it somehow happened naturally.

Egg donation

Nicola has been on the other side of the infertility spectrum. She is one of the minority of women who donate eggs for women who do not ovulate or are unable to use their own eggs.

Commerce in genetic materials is banned in Britain but, as in most areas of life, some find loopholes in the law. In 1996 it was reported in the broadsheets that some egg providers such as single mothers were being paid up to £850 per egg by traders.

For some couples, the only chance of having a baby is if another woman donates eggs; examples of women so affected are those who have had some types of cancer treatment, or a very early menopause. The number of egg donors available is pitifully small (donated sperm is less of a problem). This is probably for a number of reasons – possibly women identify more strongly with their own idea of genetic material, while the actual donation of eggs is an invasive and uncomfortable if not painful procedure. It takes a great degree of altruism to go through a surgical procedure for a woman you don't know, and there are the usual ethical considerations to think about, too.

Nicola explained how she became an egg donor.

Nicola
I read in a woman's magazine about a 26-year-old woman who had an early menopause but desperately wanted children. She put out an appeal for possible donors. After counselling, I was given drugs over a two-week period to stimulate the ovaries to produce eggs. I had six eggs first time I donated and 39 eggs the second time.

I feel that fertility treatment should be available on the NHS; infertility is not something we bring on ourselves; children are something we take for granted yet others are denied. As I have three sons myself, I obviously cannot feel that desperate sense of wanting a baby that I have often heard about, but I think I can appreciate the frustration.

Nicola had no reservations on ethical grounds.

I feel strongly about helping the recipients. My initial concern was about using some of the eggs for research, but as my nephew suffers from Duchenne muscular dystrophy I would welcome any breakthrough into the causes of such terrible diseases.

When I donated, I felt on top of the world. On coming round from the general anaesthetic at the second donation, the nurses brought me in Moët champagne and a thank you card, but best of all was a thank you card from the recipient who eventually became pregnant from one of my eggs – her grateful words reduced me to tears. I just hope that more donors come forward, as the waiting time for an attempt at treatment is approximately two years long – two years too long.

Nicola's donations have been successful.

The birth of one of my successes is imminent, while a baby boy (7½lb [3.4 kilos]) was born recently. The parents are besotted, and in a letter to me the mother has emphasised that the baby is wholly hers – of which I'm glad. Before donating I felt an unbelievable yearning to help these people; during treatment I suffered a lot of discomfort and the physical side effects of the drugs contributed to a feeling of slight ill health; afterwards I felt relief, but also frustration that I was unable to see the recipients face to face just to say I was thinking of them.

I have proudly told everybody I know and the response of everybody has been, 'I couldn't do it.' Women aren't prepared to go through so much without benefiting from it. If only they really thought of the rewards – it's a gift of life and it feels great. People tell me how brave I am, but they (mostly men) seem to have questions concerning the morals and ethics of it. Men often call it 'playing God' – well, if God has denied these people, why not? My husband has expressed his concerns because of the discomfort I felt and also he seems to think that in ten years' time the medical profession will say, 'We shouldn't have done this.' However, his support has been brilliant and he was happy to have me do this.

Nicola has one reservation: 'I'd love to follow the pregnancy through and find out more, but as it's anonymous, it would be difficult. I just want to know that all is well and the result of the birth.'

An egg donor has to be over 18 years old but under 36, obviously fertile and unafraid of the treatment: there will be several blood tests (for hepatitis B, AIDS, etc.) and drugs are given by injection before the actual donation takes place.

Another egg donor wrote as follows

I am 23 years old and I have a five-year-old daughter named Charlotte. I had Charlotte when I was 18 and when she was four weeks old her father and I separated. About 18 months later I met my new husband, Jake, and we married one year later. Charlotte now goes to full-time school and I work full-time as a retail supervisor, which I really enjoy.

Last year I read an article about a woman who was not able to conceive. She had asked if there would be any women kind enough to donate their eggs to give herself and others the chance to have children. I thought about it and discussed it with my husband. I decided to donate.

I telephoned the hospital and they sent me some details about infertility treatment and what donating would involve. After reading this I telephoned the hospital again to arrange an appointment to discuss things further.

On the day of the appointment Charlotte and I caught the train to London. I spoke to a counsellor about the operation and I was asked why I wanted to do it. I was also to have an HIV test. The treatment and respect we got from the hospital were fantastic. Charlotte was given a box of continental chocolates for 'being a good girl', which pleased us both.

A few weeks later I was given the all-clear on my HIV test and was asked if I still wanted to donate. No pressure was put on me at all and I was told that I could drop out at any time.

I was sent some hormone drugs to increase the number of eggs I produced. I had to 'sniff' a hormone from a nasal spray twice a day and I also had to inject each day, which various people did for me. The first one was done at my GP's surgery, but that was too inconvenient. My husband did the next, but felt he couldn't do any more so the rest were given to me by my Mum and a work colleague, who were both extremely proud of what I was doing. The last one had to be given at midnight the night before my next appointment at the hospital, so I took a taxi to casualty and the nurse there was very happy to give it to me.

The next morning Charlotte and I went down to London again and I had a scan of my womb to see how many eggs I had produced. The total count was 13. I was then asked to come back in ten days' time to give the eggs a chance to move to the right place and I would be operated on. I was told that on the morning of the operation I would have to be at the hospital at 9am, which I wouldn't be able to do unless I stayed in London the night before. The hospital booked a room for myself and a friend at a hotel down the road. Even at this point it was stressed to me that I could still drop out if I wanted to.

The morning before the operation my Mum, Charlotte and I caught the train to London, then took a cab to our hotel and left our belongings. We then spent the day shopping, eating and visiting museums, etc.

At around 8.45am the next day we walked to the hospital and I was booked into a room that had a telephone, TV and en suite bathroom. The atmosphere was very relaxing. I was visited by a nurse who asked me to undress and put on a hospital gown. She then explained to me what the operation involved. I don't know how long I was in theatre, but I was awoken back in my room with my Mum and Charlotte there. I felt very sick and grotty and I was told to stay in bed as long as I wanted to. The nurse suggested I had a bath and some food, but I felt too sick.

A nurse came and told me that they had successfully taken two eggs. They didn't take any more than that because the others weren't mature enough. I was also told that a lady was booked in for the next day to have my eggs, which was nice to know. At around 4pm, after I had been sick several times, we caught a cab to the station and went home.

The next day the egg donation coordinator from the hospital phoned me to see how I was feeling. A few weeks later she rang me again to tell me that the lady who had my eggs was pregnant, which made everything worthwhile.

To sum up, the experience didn't cost anything as all our expenses were paid. I didn't gain anything except the satisfaction of knowing that a lady will soon be giving birth to a baby (or maybe twins), all thanks to my eggs and the wonderful staff at the Lister Hospital, London.

People considering egg donation can contact the National Egg and Embryo Donation Society (NEEDS) on 0161 276 6000. At the current time, donors are not paid except for reasonable travelling expenses.

Some couples have qualms about using donated eggs, or sperm for that matter, as the baby is not 100 per cent genetically theirs. Kate Cargreaves described her feelings in her book, *Journey to our Children* (see p. 168). Andrea felt that 'it was very difficult having someone else's baby inside me'. She and her husband found the concept of a donor egg very difficult to come to terms with, despite it being the only option available – Andrea had been rendered infertile by cancer treatment and her own frozen eggs, removed before the treatment, did not survive the thawing out process. Hospitals where such donations take place do try very hard to match the mother and the donor in such situations, in terms of age, eye and hair colour, weight, height, skin colour, marital status and job.

The National Infertility Awareness Campaign (NIAC) is currently campaigning for infertility treatment to be available across the country in a more equitable manner, so that everyone has access to treatment. King's College Hospital Assisted Conception Unit Patient Support Group (KACUPSG) in association with CHILD have recently run a massive egg donation campaign, catching media attention with provocative billboards in London and the South East, calling for women to donate their eggs to help childless couples trying for a family. The campaign was launched in response to the current national critical shortage of egg donors and the poster ran the bold question: 'Are You the Kind of Woman who Could Make Another Woman Pregnant?' Again, contact NEEDS if you are interested.

The HFEA and the Royal College of Nursing have both set up working parties to investigate the issues surrounding egg and sperm donation in response to the urgency felt by couples waiting to conceive. An estimated one in six couples seek medical assistance to achieve a pregnancy at some time during their reproductive lives.

Many people remain uncomfortable about egg donation (although less ado is made about sperm donation). The charity LIFE feels that it is ethically and practically full of problems, pointing to the fact that women who have their children adopted often suffer regret and loss and search for their children in later life. The same feelings could apply to egg donors. A national newspaper criticised the campaign for making egg donation seem like a public duty, rather like blood donation, and expressed the view that the HFEA should have sought to have the campaign halted. There is a great depth of feeling, not about fertility treatment per se but certainly about using donors to make that treatment possible.

The Patients' Association has also expressed its reservations about such a campaign, noting that egg donation is a serious procedure and that women need to be very carefully counselled before going ahead. A number of newspaper commentators looked back to the great frozen embryo debate of 1996, when 3,300 human embryos, retrieved for but not ultimately used in the process of assisted conception, were destroyed after five years. The argument is that in many artificial conceptions there will be a surplus of embryos – not all eggs retrieved are implanted, because of the risk of multiple pregnancies. These spare embryos can be frozen for future use, destroyed or experimented upon – although it is illegal to experiment on embryos over 14 days old, or to attempt cloning or production of embryos by combining the egg or sperm of humans with that of animals.

In Ireland the problem is avoided as no more than three eggs are fertilised at any one time, but this possibly reduces the chances of a successful pregnancy. But the question of the ownership and future of genetic material remains a running sore in the infertility arena.

A leading broadsheet newspaper ran a recent article on the benefits of egg sharing. This is a scheme whereby couples going through the IVF process donate spare eggs (acquired through the use of ovary-stimulating drugs) to couples who need egg donation to begin infertility treatment. Dr Kamal Ajuha, the scientific director of the Cromwell IVF centres, who has pioneered egg sharing in Britain, estimates that there are at least 2,000 women in the country awaiting donor eggs. Egg sharing has clear benefits over straightforward egg donation: first, the eggs are only available through the help of medicine, so the donation is less intrusive and perhaps less emotive; second, the logic of egg sharing is obvious, as two desperate groups – those who need donated eggs and those who require standard IVF – can help each other.

The usual practice is that, in exchange for the eggs, the recipient normally pays for the donor's IVF treatment and drugs. Dr Ajuha thus describes the scheme as 'pragmatic altruism' and he adds, 'I believe it is the only ethical way forward for egg donation programmes in this country, because it involves a form of generosity which is closer to the reality of human nature than the purely unselfish anonymous donation of eggs.' He is very uneasy about moves by the HFEA to phase out egg sharing on the grounds that it is a form of 'payment in kind' to donors, leaving purely altruistic donation as the only form of egg donation permitted. Sam Abdalla, director of the IVF unit at the Lister Hospital in London, which has one of Britain's largest and most successful egg-donation programmes, says that he personally would like very much to introduce the egg-sharing scheme. He is reluctant to do so, however, because the HFEA appears set to phase out the practice. 'There is a high degree of hypocrisy about the idea of payment in kind', he is quoted in the national press as saying:

> The facts are that 99 per cent of NHS clinics are charging patients for their IVF treatment. If a patient has no money left, this form of treatment means that you have a chance of having a baby if you are prepared to share your eggs. Egg-sharing is about two women who are essentially in need of each other.

A final word on egg donation from a kind contributor.

Anon

My husband and I have been trying to start a family for five and a half years. As with most couples, we have been through interminable investigations, starting with our very helpful GP, progressing to seeing a local gynaecologist (using my private health insurance from work), and eventually moving to a private hospital which offers assisted conception services and funding the expense ourselves, albeit with some initial help from the GP for drugs through the NHS. It seems that I am suffering from ovulatory problems although no firm conclusion has ever been reached, which is frustrating in itself.

We are a very lucky couple who have a good, strong relationship and very supportive friends. We both have good jobs, a beautiful house in a friendly village. None of this has eliminated our pain, but I believe that our relationship has become stronger because of the trials we have been through.

Initially, we were both embarrassed to talk about the matter – even with each other to begin with. We were scared to admit that there could be anything wrong. Everything else we had ever done had worked out, so why not this? I was more concerned than my husband at this stage and read *Getting Pregnant* by Robert [Professor Lord] Winston avidly and repeatedly. I have since read several other books, joined CHILD and ISSUE [patient support groups] and attended various conferences on infertility. Being able to go away and learn about the problems and treatments has helped me to cope with the seesaw of my emotions and enabled me to understand better what and why certain actions are suggested. I think we have got used to the problem and are more able to talk about it. A difficult decision is when/if to tell work. I think we timed our revelation just right, and this has made it a little easier to incorporate our treatment into our working lives.

We were both terrified of becoming one of those sad couples we were vaguely aware of for whom getting a baby is the sole occupation in life. Apart from anything else, we felt that this would be detrimental to our chances of success, so we were conscious of trying to strike the right balance, taking the matter seriously but not forgetting that we have each other and a whole life going on which we should try to maintain.

It was difficult to start the ball rolling by going to see our GP, and I was fairly strong in pushing my husband to make the first appointment in order to ensure that he felt as strongly about the matter as I did. Our doctor immediately organised some preliminary tests after first asking why we hadn't come sooner than the nine months we'd waited.

The infertility unit I am attending believes my best (only) course of action is to go for egg donation. This is not only more complex but also more expensive and there is a desperate shortage of egg donors. The waiting list for donors is quoted as being approximately ten months, but significantly shorter if you bring a donor with you. I was also told that the donor should be anonymous. I know the donor is not allowed to benefit financially from the donation, which to me seems a bit crazy – I'm sure some kind of financial recognition should be offered for the not inconsiderable inconvenience she has to go through in order to make a donation. Of course this should not be such a large sum as to make it the sole reason for somebody offering to donate.

I tried to find potential donors, and indeed some of my friends had already said (when they didn't know it would come to it) that they would like to help if they could. Donating an egg involves very careful monitoring and counselling; out of those who make an initial approach to the hospital only two out of ten actually end up making a donation. My sister was one of the people who offered to try to help, but she felt very strongly that she would like to donate directly to me (not an anonymous donation). I must admit that I also feel that if I have to have a donated egg, then one from the same genetic pool would be my favoured option. To my amazement, when she raised this with the hospital, they said it was possible although our case would have to go before the Ethics Committee and we would have to have very careful counselling. We have been successful with this and are now nearly at the stage of egg collection.

Adoption

For couples who find they are unable to have children of their own, adoption may clearly be an alternative. It is vital that any decision to pursue this course is taken by both partners. The matter of childlessness must have been thoroughly discussed and accepted by both of the involved parties, and it is essential to feel that an adopted child could be loved just as a natural-born child would be. The British Agencies for Adoption and Fostering (BAAF) in London are there to help. Very few babies are available for adoption these days, and therefore the adoption agencies have extremely strict criteria for prospective parents – age, marital status and health are all taken into account, and usually babies are only offered for adoption to infertile couples who have clearly come to terms with their infertility. Couples are unlikely to be considered if they are undergoing investigation or treatment and therefore still hoping to conceive.

Hazel

Our experience of infertility has been over the past 21 years. I was on the pill when we married in 1972 and three years later we decided to start a family. When nothing happened after one year we approached our doctor, who referred us to a specialist.

Over the next ten years we endured every possible test going and were seen at three hospitals. The worst part was having to sit in the waiting rooms with pregnant women or new mothers with their babies.

Eventually we were told that they could find nothing wrong with either of us and they could not help us any further. At this point we decided to try IVF and were referred to Hallam Medical Centre in London. Our first appointment was in 1987.

During the next two years we had twelve attempts at IVF. Our last attempt was in January 1989. In 1991 we decided to try to adopt two older children. We were successful and Matthew and Samantha moved in with us in May 1993. They were legally adopted in June 1994.

Looking back I realise just how obsessed we were with the IVF treatments. We were spending thousands of pounds and never batted an eyelid. Before each treatment we were actually looking forward to my period starting so we could start the programme. The travelling to and from the clinic for daily scans, blood tests and injections was quite stressful. Some of the injections I managed to do at home myself. Our doctor was very understanding (and fascinated by the whole thing) and let us have all the drugs on prescription.

Having IVF was quite traumatic and we didn't tell our family or friends because we couldn't handle the questions like 'When are you going to make us grandparents?', which would have put more pressure on us.

During each IVF treatment, and especially when it failed, I would say, 'That's it. I can't take any more,' and the strain of the last two weeks, waiting to see if it had been successful, was probably worse than the actual treatment. After the disappointment had been forgotten, I was always so eager to have one last try. It was like gambling. We would always think that this was the time we would hit the jackpot.

After twelve attempts and because I was 37 and the odds were not good, we decided to call it a day. Afterwards I was surprised at the relief I felt.

We are glad that we tried everything and went through so much to have a family. If we had accepted childlessness and done nothing we would have regretted it. At least now we can look back and say that at least we tried.

'They' say the worst stress is caused by moving house, divorce or changing jobs. Well, 'they' obviously have not tried starting a family.

Another couple among our contributors, Sarah and her husband, were married twelve years ago and, after trying to conceive for three years, realised that they might need some medical intervention. They underwent tests and it was discovered that Sarah had scar tissue in her tubes. Sarah was enormously impressed and touched by the kindness and efficiency shown by her GP and, on medical advice, had laser treatment. Sarah knows that her husband, a traditional male, thought it was easier that it was she who was the 'one with the problem' – he would have found it much harder to cope with a fertility issue of his own. The couple have supported each other throughout, largely by discussing every small issue and not hiding any of their innermost feelings.

When IVF was first discussed, she and her husband made a firm decision that they would have three attempts and then stop. No NHS treatment was available, but they had the funds and were happy to be able to try IVF, although they recognised from the outset that their chances of success were slim.

Sarah used the same medical unit for each of her three IVF attempts, and felt that as time went by, and demands upon the facility were greater, the service became less personal. For example, on her first visits she was provided with a private room and attended to on a one-to-one basis. By her third treatment, however, she was expected to stay on a small ward with three other women and she would have much preferred her own privacy, since she found the whole experience extremely traumatic.

Two years ago, Sarah and her husband took the brave step to stick to their initial decision and recognise that they would not give birth naturally. They are still relatively young – Sarah is 34 and her husband 36. No counselling was offered, but Sarah felt in any case that she must come to terms with her childlessness in her own way. She felt strongly supported by a friend of the family who has also suffered from infertility and has adopted children, and was free to talk to this friend at length. Sarah and her husband put their names down on the local authority adoption list eight years ago and are hopeful that, fairly soon, they will be offered a baby. Interestingly, the county list has now been closed: it is just so rare for babies to become available that the service is being withdrawn.

We asked Sarah what messages she would want to pass on to future sufferers. She feels that it is important to recognise from the outset that the chances are very slim, and that the easiest way to cope is to be open and honest with everyone you meet – pretending that your childlessness is voluntary simply adds an unnecessary pressure to what is already a very difficult emotion. Sarah also commented on the 1996 BBC1 television series *Making Babies* saying that such programmes are wonderful in that they remove some of the dreadful taboos which society has left us with. She feels that the more recognition infertility has, the easier it becomes to admit that you too are a victim.

Surrogacy

Surrogate mothering is surrounded by controversy, although it is in evidence in the Bible (where Abraham's infertile wife begged him to have a child by their servant). The major objections are twofold: first, an objection to the 'selling' of babies in those instances where money changes hands; and, second, the likelihood of the surrogate mother changing her mind after the birth – and the related difficulties of 'ownership'.

There follows a fascinating insight into surrogacy by a mother involved first-hand.

Kathy, happily married with two daughters (aged eleven and six), offered herself as a surrogate mother to a couple (Carol and

Andrew) whom she met through COTS. As Carol had a hysterectomy following cervical cancer, but can still produce eggs, Kathy planned to be a host surrogate (that is, a fertilised embryo from the other couple would be implanted into her uterus) as opposed to a 'straight' surrogate (using her own eggs and Andrew's sperm via artificial insemination). There have so far been two failed attempts at implantation.

COTS recommends a 'compensation rate' for surrogates to cover expenses, time off work, money for clothes and equipment and travel, and to compensate the family of the host mother for her time and effort. It is clear that Kathy was not completely comfortable with this, especially as she formed an ever closer bond with the other parents. She wrote as follows.

Kathy

The news has been on today, with the professor from our clinic in the news again. Apparently he is putting patients in touch with an organisation called HOPE, who put people in touch with egg donors. The trouble is that HOPE's donors are charging £850 to donate. Also the clinic charges £250, and our professor charges £4,000 to do the business. It is extortionate. I donated eggs in 1992 and I did it because I felt it was the right thing to do, not for financial gain. I didn't receive a penny, and wouldn't want to ... It doesn't cost £10,000 to have a baby for someone else, and I shall probably end up doing it for nothing as Carol and Andrew are my friends and having got to know them so well over the past eight months I feel really bad about wanting 'compensation'. It was only the figure recommended by COTS (apparently that is the 'going rate'). But I think I will leave it to Carol and Andrew to give me a sum at the end. As long as they pay me a monthly figure while I am not earning at my job. It should be their decision to pay me what they can afford.

Later ...

Andrew and I talked about money and Andrew said we must stick to the agreement and payment must be made for time off work and expenses. I explained I wasn't doing it because I wanted the money, and they are now our friends, but he said he doesn't want to offend me but must pay.

Kathy also became very angry about being misled by their London clinic. In the first egg collection from Carol, seven eggs were retrieved. Three were implanted and the other four were described as being of lesser quality, but were frozen anyway. The clinic said it was worth doing because it was free. However, the eggs disintegrated on thawing – leading to a major disappointment to the surrogate mother and parents, who were all prepared for implantation. There was varying opinion from specialists at the clinic. Some said the eggs should never have been frozen. This inconsistency caused much upset. There was also divided opinion as to whether the host surrogate should be implanted according to her natural cycle, or should use drugs to control her cycle so that she was ready for implantation immediately after the eggs were taken from Carol. The parents/surrogates badly needed the comfort of knowing that professional opinion was undivided. Kathy wrote:

April 1996. Carol and Andrew went to London for a consultation. Carol told the consultant that every time they go they see someone different, and that a lot of mistakes have been made – like freezing their four embryos when really they were not fit for freezing, and then to build our hopes up and get me ready for a transfer only to be disappointed when they did not survive. The bad news is that from January 1996 it has been law to freeze either embryos or sperm for at least six months. This means that since we have nothing frozen, we cannot go ahead with another try until November 1996. If only they had told us this in January, then we could have saved four months. Carol has really got no time to lose since she has been told that when you have a hysterectomy, your ovaries start packing up and three years after the operation is when they start to deteriorate – her operation was two years ago, so time is not on our side. Anyway, there is nothing we can do but wait until November and pray that it works the third time.

The most recent news is that a third attempt had resulted in a positive pregnancy test, but the embryos were not strong enough to survive. Kathy hopes that they will not give up yet.

In America there is a Centre for Surrogate Parenting and Egg Donation in Beverly Hills. The cost of surrogacy in the USA is around £30,000, but in the UK, while surrogacy goes on, it is unregulated – which often leads to further heartache when a contract breaks down. In surrogacy cases where the birth mother hosts an embryo supplied by a woman who cannot bear her own child, such breakdowns can lead to a situation of particular loss for the genetic mother who loses all contact with the baby. In the UK the loophole providing for open-ended 'legitimate expenses' means surrogates may be paid anything from £10,000 to £100,000.

Unexplained assistance

All gynaecologists can tell stories of patients who become naturally pregnant, against all expectations, during their fertility treatment. This occurs most commonly at two junctures: the first when the patient is initially offered treatment and put on a waiting list; the second when all forms of treatment have failed and the patient comes to terms with childlessness. It is believed, but unproven, that in both of these circumstances the patient psychologically relaxes, and perhaps in this way creates a hormonal environment in which conception can finally occur. These natural pregnancies do not appear in the statistics of the fertility unit – but perhaps they should ...

Glenys
We have one daughter who was born after five years of trying. After she was born we decided to let nature take its course, but two and a half years later nothing had happened so we started trying with medical assistance. It was a time of waiting, trying fertility drugs, trying different combinations – all with no success. IVF was our next and only option. We felt that if we tried IVF, whether it worked or not, then at least we had tried. We were accepted for IVF. We were given the list of drugs to get, the times and dates of tests, scans and drug administration. The treatment wasn't too bad. I'd had so many blood tests etc. in the past that I felt a few more didn't matter.

We succeeded in getting through all the stages of IVF and had three embryos implanted. The next two weeks were the most important. They were also the longest and toughest weeks we ever went through. Time went so slowly, but I felt that as long as I wasn't bleeding there was hope.

The time came for the test. Still no bleeding. I was really hoping for a positive result. The result was negative. We were very upset and I cried for the whole weekend.

I decided to pamper myself a bit and went for acupuncture and aromatherapy. The lady I went to knew what I had been through and concentrated on massaging my tummy and lower back to bring fresh blood and oxygen to the reproductive area. My period arrived and I just got on with my life, still having massage every two weeks or so. At one massage I told her she was really hurting my lower back. She said that a large area was inflamed. My next period was due around this time.

A week later I did a pregnancy test and got the shock of my life when it turned out positive. I was stunned. The first thing I did after telling my husband was ring the IVF unit. They couldn't have been nicer to me. They took care of me until I was twelve weeks pregnant and at that stage everything was progressing well. I had a lovely time being pregnant and morning, noon and night sickness was very welcome indeed.

In January 1996 I delivered my second daughter, seven and a half years after my first. She is a most beautiful baby and I can't let her out of my sight yet as I can't believe how lucky I am to have her. I believe that the IVF had something to do with my becoming pregnant as I had IVF in January and was pregnant in April. The IVF unit told me that this happens in a good few cases. I am so glad that I was one of the few.

Secondary infertility

The inability to conceive following an earlier pregnancy is generally not viewed sympathetically by others, but the frustration and sadness are no different from those associated with primary infertility. Many individuals feel that those lucky enough to have a child (or even to be able to conceive without assistance) should feel guilty at using up resources if they want another child.

If you can conceive but not carry babies to term, then you are suffering from secondary, not primary infertility. Sometimes secondary infertility is the continuation of primary infertility, or it may be unexpected and new. Ask any parent with two or more children and you will discover that each child is equally wanted and loved – it follows that every child attempted by a sufferer of secondary infertility is also greatly wanted. Because you have one child already, you may also suffer added problems – your child will be viewed as an only child and you will be constantly asked if you plan more children.

Acceptance of childlessness

It would not be complete to close this chapter without reference to those who make the positive decision that their own answer to infertility is to accept the diagnosis and follow their lives in other directions.

Alison
I had known since my teens that it was unlikely I would ever have children, and I found myself reluctant to form relationships as I grew older, afraid of discovering that no one wanted a sterile woman.

When I finally met Bill, I knew that I wanted to marry him, and so I told him very early on that I would probably never have kids. He has been endlessly supportive and has never even suggested treatment. Once, when I timidly told him about a friend of mine at work who was having IVF, he said, 'I would support you in every way if you wanted something like that, but just do what you feel comfortable with.'

I often think it must almost be easier for me to accept than it is for him, because I have had so long to get used to the idea – I did my mourning when I was 15 years old. Perhaps that's why I've never really considered IVF treatment, because early on I came to terms with a life without children and managed very successfully to convince myself that there are worse things to lose than the potential of children.

Bill and I neither avoid other people's children, nor go out of our way to spend time with them. I honestly think that our life is full and happy. We share many hobbies and sometimes one of us will admit that if we had kids we would not be able to indulge ourselves nearly as much as we do.

Families are great, but so is life without them.

Jilly
My husband and I married in our mid-20s and waited over five years before we decided that, if we were going to have children, then the time was right to do so. We had both always assumed that we would, at some point, have children, but had never discussed it as our life's goal.

The discovery of our infertility came as a real shock and, as so often happens, the knowledge that I couldn't have children made me suddenly want them desperately.

We were told that IVF was our only option (my tubes were irrevocably damaged), and that it could be a long, stressful and expensive procedure. There was a three-year waiting list in our area, and the only financial help we could expect was for the drugs involved.

I went immediately to begin the process to get our names on the waiting list. My husband and I both earned reliable salaries, but we had no savings, so I began to investigate sources of money (family, mainly). I became absolutely obsessed with the idea of using IVF to provide me with the children I now wanted so badly. I refused to book a summer holiday, preferring to save the money and plan the nursery. I made Christmas a misery, crying about having no little feet to patter around and endlessly re-reading the IVF documentation. I ignored my husband and retreated within myself.

It was two years along the line before I was brought to my senses. My husband, a gentle and kind man, reached the end of his tether. He sat me down and explained that our life before conception had been wonderful in his eyes. He reminded me of the fun we had had, the great times we had spent, just the two of us. He told me that all he had ever wanted was to be part of my life, and that if there were to be no children to grace that life, then that was a loss, but one that he could bear. He told me that he would give the earth to return me to the funny, loving wife that he used to live with. I was knocked off my feet. I realised that all along I had been subconsciously convinced that my infertility had been something he would hold against me, and that I had to find a way to redress the balance. I was sure that he would love me properly only if I could give him a child. Suddenly to understand that he would love me most if I stopped thinking about children was a revelation to me. I cried for almost 24 hours and, at the end of that, I was almost myself again.

We removed our name from the IVF list and comforted ourselves that this gesture alone meant that another couple would get to the top sooner. We took a three-week holiday and laughed like drains. Don't get me wrong, the pain didn't die – I still looked at complete families and felt a sense of isolation and emptiness, but I knew now that the best path forward for us was just to enjoy what we had and try to make the most of life.

I am now postmenopausal, and in a funny way that makes me content. My marriage is sound, and I know that the IVF route would probably have lost me a loving husband.

Life is different without children – I can see that by comparing my life to those around me who have completed their families. But it needn't be worse. We have fun, we have friends and we have each other.

7 The lottery of IVF

Acceptance on to funded IVF programmes seems to occur at a widely varying rate around the country. Some health authorities will not fund any IVF treatment; others will fund only one attempt; others still will fund up to three. Some authorities will not consider NHS IVF if the couple are also trying private treatment. The variation seems unfair and the criteria appear to be arbitrary. There has been a great deal of criticism in the media of clinics treating 'unsuitable' candidates: people who are seen as socially rather than biologically unsuitable. There has also been bad publicity about age limits. Most IVF clinics now refuse treatment to women over the age of 40 – some refuse women over 35 – based on the rationale of scarce resources meaning a line has to be drawn. There is also a severe shortage of egg donors, who are more likely to be required with women of this age group. Private clinics, however, may set their own age limits, and some choose 50 years as a cut-off point. The HFEA, which licenses both NHS and private infertility clinics, does not lay down any age guidelines.

Fertility problems in women multiply after the age of 35, and once a woman is 37 she will produce fewer eggs. Those which she does produce are more susceptible to genetic mutations. Generally, parents wanting babies want perfect ones, so age can lead to another ethical problem – that of genetic screening and destruction of a non-perfect embryo at the very earliest stages of life.

Almost all of the people we questioned in the course of research for this book felt strongly about the issue of age and its relevance to fertility treatment, but opinion was divided. Sympathy was, on the whole, on the side of women over the age of 30. Many interviewees believed that fewer resources should be channelled towards younger candidates, in the belief that medical abilities will continue to develop rapidly over the next ten years, so those people still in their 20s today will have the opportunity to benefit from scientific advancements in future years.

The issue of age is also intrinsically linked with that of experience and maturity. It is widely felt that a couple in the first flush of marriage may not have the experience to deal with the inevitable stress brought about by fertility treatment.

On the other side of the coin, there is also a strongly held belief that parents giving birth for the first time in their 50s should ask themselves some very stern questions about their ability to be fully active and contributing parents.

A number of ethical issues have raised themselves in recent years. Pauline Lyon, aged 52, is the oldest woman in Britain to have combined IVF with egg donation – she allegedly lied about her age. Other cases have included Mary Shearing, an American who in 1992 became the oldest mother of test tube twins at 53 years. Likewise, in 1994 a 62-year-old Sicilian woman gave birth after being artificially inseminated with her husband's sperm a year after he died, and Professor Severino Antinori received a good deal of criticism for treating a British woman who was pregnant at the age of 63.

Should there be imposed age limits – if so, where should these be set? Postmenopausal women are likely to need egg donation, which is in short supply. Is there an argument for offering such eggs to younger women and those without any children? Some critics point to the evidence that older parents may make better parents – and older these days is young in comparison to women in their 50s some decades ago; women tend to be healthier, for example. It could also be argued that many women become pregnant naturally in their 40s, so why should the opportunity be denied to those who need assistance?

Some health authorities are introducing distinguishing measures for couples wanting assisted conception treatments. For example, in 1996 a report mentioned that funding for treatment from Wigan and Bolton Health Authority stood at a static level of £50,000. Couples in these areas are not being accepted on to waiting lists until the lists have substantially decreased in size, which for many could mean a five-year wait to get on the list. Desperate financial situations seem to call for desperate measures. It is difficult to decide who should have treatment under a rationing system, but this health authority has laid down certain criteria for people who will be new to the waiting list. The authority says that the criteria are based upon clinical judgement, but some would argue strongly that in fact they are social criteria. They include two main points:

1. Smokers who refuse to attend smoking cessation sessions will not be eligible for conception treatments. Arguably, the welfare of the child and chances of continuing a pregnancy to term are issues here as the detrimental effects of smoking on pregnancy are well documented.
2. Those who have had a child from a previous relationship or have previously been funded for subfertility treatment will also not be accepted.

In some areas health authorities have ceased all funding for assisted conception services, arguing a poor success rate. The cost of treatment varies, but in 1996 one cycle of treatment could cost up to £5,000. IVF could cost £1,600–2,400 per cycle. For those who already have children, this may seem a good deal of money set aside to deal with non-life-threatening cases, so there is often little sympathy in the public mind about the needs of childless people.

To compound the funding difficulties, recent reports have highlighted disputes between health authorities and GPs over who pays for the fertility drugs childless couples need. Many health authorities will fund one cycle of IVF, but will not finance the drugs which stimulate a woman's ovaries and are a prerequisite for treatment.

Many GPs (who also have budgets to work to) deny responsibility for the drugs, seeing them as part of hospital treatment. The cost of the drugs (£600–800 in 1996) is not inconsiderable, and the main beneficiaries appear to be drugs companies who charge such inflated prices. If health authorities do pick up the tab, then rationing necessarily has to occur somewhere else – as successive governments constantly remind us, NHS funding is not a bottomless pit.

Back in 1993, about half of all health authorities in the United Kingdom did not provide even the most basic NHS fertility treatment. In April 1996 genetically engineered FSH (follicle-stimulating hormone) became available, but this is even more expensive (25–50 per cent more than the drugs derived from the urine of pre-menopausal women). If infertility is a medical condition, then it should be treated as one, but increasingly health authorities view it as a social or personal problem and there is little consensus. Responsibility is hard to pinpoint.

GPs are in a difficult position too. According to Department of Health guidelines, they should not prescribe drugs unless they take clinical responsibility (look at the brouhaha in 1996 over Mandy Allwood, who carried octuplets and miscarried them all), but the drugs needed are actually part of intensive hospital treatment where the GP has no control. Fertility treatment is not considered by the British Medical Association to be a 'core service' or a treatment which GPs are obliged to provide. GPs remain reluctant to fund treatment because of costs and for clinical reasons; the result is a Catch 22 situation for the couples involved. It poses a complex medico-legal problem, one of many which arise from infertility treatment (such as what to do with frozen embryos). Should we take money from primary care and give it to sufferers of infertility? Few of the fertile are likely to be sympathetic.

Wendy, aged 27 and Richard, 24, have been trying for a baby for five years. They are now one year through a three-year waiting list for IVF on the NHS. Wendy's problem started with a miscarriage at ten weeks.

Wendy

I was sent to hospital and kept in overnight as I was bleeding a lot. I was scanned and told everything had come away, so I didn't need a D&C. After that, however, I had bad problems with my periods – they were happening every two to three weeks, and were heavy. Eighteen months later I moved and a new doctor sent me to hospital, where I had a D&C. The hospital didn't do anything else but referred me on to St Mary's. They tested my fallopian tubes by injecting an opaque fluid into them; this was very painful. They also checked Richard's sperm count. The first time round it was low, but second time and thereafter it was OK. About a year ago they investigated me with a camera but couldn't see any problem; everything seemed fine. I felt like I was back to square one after all this time. There were no blocked tubes or anything. My hormones were imbalanced, they thought, and I was put on Clomid to produce more eggs but it just made me really moody. I was accepted as a candidate for IVF.

Wendy works with babies in her capacity as a nursery nurse:

Sometimes it can really get to you. Everybody around me at the moment is pregnant. One friend has two children already and is pregnant again – it was an accident; she's not bothered. People don't like to tell me when they're pregnant, but I am open about the problem as lots of people ask me why I've no children. A friend had a baby recently and I was really upset.

The couple don't allocate blame:

Richard lives for today – he says if we were supposed to have children, then we'd have them. We have considered adoption, but have made the decision not to investigate it until after IVF. I now want to try an ovulation kit to see what happens. The hospital has said to relax and not think about it, but all the time I'm in an environment where I can see mums and babies; I also see young women with babies who don't really want them. At least in my work I can give my love to other children because I can't have them. I get very attached to the children I work with.

When the hospital first suggested IVF, Wendy wasn't keen:

When she first said I'll put you on IVF, I wasn't happy about it because I didn't agree with messing around with my body if there's a natural way, but Richard agreed that we should put our names down and if anything happens in the meantime, that's great. We've tried temperature charts, everything. Richard's been very supportive. I've asked him if he'd stay with me if I couldn't have children – he says he wouldn't leave me because of that. Sometimes, I'm sure the entire medical profession in Manchester has seen my private parts.

Unlike many couples, Wendy feels their sex life has not been badly affected. .

We were advised by the hospital to make love once a week to allow Richard's sperm count to build up. The desire to make babies hasn't taken over – to begin with, every time my period came I felt depressed and down, but now I've moved on from that. But I get fed up with the waiting. When I had hormone tablets, I could have killed. I asked the doctor what the side effects were – he mentioned depression, insomnia and personality disorders. My body seemed totally confused. I'm so glad I don't take them now, but I hate the sitting and waiting.

Wendy doesn't want to face the idea of being childless: 'I don't know how I'd cope with being childless. I'm still hoping. I'll go as far as I can to have a baby.'

Like most infertile couples, Wendy has had her fair share of insensitive comments:

> People say, 'Don't worry, there's plenty of time, you're young, etc.' Well, they're not in my shoes are they? They're not desperate to have children; they don't understand. My mother says we can't afford a baby and it's a horrible world anyway, but I'd go without anything to provide my baby with what was needed. My sister has two children – it makes me feel as if I'm inadequate and incapable. A lot of my family have died, there are few of us left, so a baby wouldn't only be for me. Supposed friends say, 'You're not pregnant yet, then; better get a move on,' when they know all we've been through – they still say it. Not knowing why is the worst bit. If only they'd found something wrong and could treat it, but to have all those tests for nothing, it just leaves me back at the beginning. The hospital staff didn't understand my feelings when they told me they could find nothing – I was just another number to them and it is just a job.

The cost of IVF is prohibitive for couples like Wendy and Richard:

> I don't understand why the waiting list is so long and why at some hospitals it's a lot shorter. Infertility treatment should be fully available on the NHS, but perhaps with an age limit, but I don't know what that limit should be. If so many people have infertility problems, why is the IVF success rate so low? Why can't they do more research if it is needed so much? People might not mind paying the money if there was more certainty. I don't think I would pay to have it done privately, because the success rate is not high enough. If it was a dead cert, I'd borrow the money from Mum, but otherwise I won't. I wouldn't take out a bank loan. It would be a major struggle to find £2,000. Some money will come to us soon from Richard's share of his Dad's house, but we won't spend it on IVF; there is not enough certainty.

While many relationships struggle under the burden of infertility, Wendy feels theirs is stronger. 'It has brought us closer together. He's very supportive. I had my cards read – they said I'd come into some money which will help me to relax and feel more financially secure, so who knows?' Wendy was unaware of support groups for childless couples, such as ISSUE, and felt there was a dearth of information available. However, she realises the risks associated with IVF pregnancy: the thought of twins or even triplets doesn't faze her.

Wendy's message for other women and her own motto is: 'Don't give up hope.'

One contributor summed up her message with real feeling.

Tracey
Hopefully one day there will be more understanding and support for infertile couples and more help with costs of treatment. When you find out you are infertile everything is left to you to research and look into. No one sits with you to explain to you options, or answers your questions. After all, when you find out you are infertile your life's dream crumbles and your heart goes on the biggest coaster ride of its life. I wish I wasn't writing this and that no one would ever have to read it, but that's life.

I can't really provide any answers; everyone is individual and will have to deal with it in their own way. Remember you are not the only one going through it, your partner and family are too. Just let their love help you and don't feel guilty if you resent others for having a baby. It is a natural feeling and deep down you wouldn't wish them to go through what you are. It is just a way of getting rid of the anger in you. I know you will worry about what other people think, but it doesn't really matter. If they don't like it or can't cope, then they don't really love you. They should love you for who you are and not what you can't give them. This applies to everything in life. Love and understanding will help dull the pain and never, never give up hope.

I have watched several different programmes on the TV about the different ways infertile couples have had children and every time you watch one it will set you off thinking in a different way. You will find the way that's best for you. Patience is all you need and one day you just may be giving that child the love you have and want to share. If you stop hoping and praying you might as well give up now. When you hold that baby or child in your arms for the first time you will know it was worth all the pain. I hope you all get what you want one day, me included.

One of our contributors kindly sent in a fact sheet for self-funding patients, produced by the Fertility Centre run by St Bartholomew's, the London and the Royal hospitals. The wording of the letter is perhaps indicative of the 1990s, offering patients 'the opportunity' to pay for their own treatment, which is charged at 'almost cost price' (that is, only very slightly more than is charged to the health authority). It also makes the point that the Fertility Centre has more capacity to treat patients than is being used – so self-funding is not queue jumping: those in the NHS queue will remain there until funded. The letter suggests that once a GP has made the referral, a letter clearly stating a wish to self-fund means the case and payment are processed quickly.

The costs of each treatment are outlined and these include everything for a cycle, except the cost of drugs (approximately £500 in 1996) which a GP may agree to fund.

We have also been provided with the following price list (also for 1996) from Bourn Hall, Cambridge:

IVF	£2,200
GIFT	£2,200
ZIFT (Zygote Intrafallopian Transfer)	£2,700
ICSI	£2,950
IVF with ICSI	£4,250
IVF with donor oocytes (underdeveloped eggs)	£4,500
IVF surrogacy	£3,100

At these prices, it is not surprising that patients not funded by their health authorities are prepared to go into huge debt to have a child. Are health trusts working in the field of infertility exploiting the desire to have children? To what extent is the biological suitability of patients for the various treatments assesssed?

International infertility legislation

The International Federation of Infertility Patients Associations (IFIPA) offers a combined platform for infertility organisations around the world. In the April 1996 issue of its magazine, *Infertility World*, it records the following information about the availability of infertility treatment in different countries.

Australia

Australian consumers are represented on the Federal Council of the Fertility Society of Australia (FSA) and on the industry accrediting body, the Reproductive Technology Accreditation Committee (RTAC). They thus have access to reliable information about treatment outcomes, possible drug side effects and the quality of service provided by individual clinics.

In 1990 the Australian prime minister recognised infertility as a medical condition and granted reimbursement of assisted reproductive technology (ART) treatment by the Australian national health scheme.

Access to government-funded drugs used in treatment in Australia is provided only to those clinics which have been accredited by RTAC, and the availability of counselling is a requirement of accreditation.

Canada

In March 1997 a Royal Commission in Canada inexplicably recommended that access to ART should be restricted to women with bilateral fallopian tube damage. One may wonder how the infertile male citizens of Canada feel about this rejection of their health-care needs.

France

In France four cycles of ART are paid for by the social security system, to a limit (in 1995) of Fr 10,000, at a number of public and private centres authorised by a national commission. A new law came into place in 1995 aiming to control ART and the following aspects shocked infertility sufferers.

1. Without consideration of women who marry at 38 years of age, the law now requires two years of conjugal life before a request for ART can be considered
2. When a donation of sperm or egg is to be used in IVF, the couple concerned have to proceed with legal formalities in front of a judge before a treatment cycle can begin. This threatens any possibility of anonymity.

Sweden

The first IVF baby was born in Sweden in 1982. In January 1989 the country passed a law that regulates IVF. This law forbids egg donations and IVF with sperm donors and surrogate motherhood. It also allows embryos to be frozen for just one year. As of 1997, a proposal is under consideration to permit egg donation and a prolongation of the freezing time for the embryos to five years. IRIS, the Swedish national patients' association, hopes that the same law will be valid in all the Scandinavian countries. Finland, for example, permits all kinds of assisted fertilisation.

Switzerland

In Switzerland, access to ART is threatened, largely because of legislation which ties together ART and genetic engineering and seeks to limit their use. It is disappointing to see such opportunistic abuse of a vulnerable segment of the community.

USA

Legislation regulating clinics has been passed in the American House of Representatives, but no funds have been allocated for its implementation. The original Clinton health-care reform plan excluded coverage for IVF, but a proposal based on Clinton's plan included comprehensive coverage (under pregnancy-related benefits). Federal legislation was adopted in summer 1996.

Ethical problems

Just as doctors were criticised widely for the prescribing of fertility drugs to Mandy Allwood (see Chapter 1), there is also criticism of the way in which Diane Blood has been treated in her mission to have her dead husband's baby (see below). It is also interesting to note how the media has dealt with the two cases. Mandy Allwood, who has been portrayed as a socially irresponsible woman who disobeyed her doctor's instructions to abstain from sexual intercourse after taking fertility drugs, is a woman with a supposedly dubious history and absentee boyfriend, who seemingly continued with a multiple pregnancy to make some big money from the press. Whether or not this is true, the case has not helped the cause of fertility treatment in the public's mind. The Mandy Allwood case added fuel to the fire of people who feel that fertility treatments need more regulation. Mandy Allwood's case developed rapid fame when it was discovered that she was pregnant with octuplets, that she refused to selectively terminate any of them, that she had apparently not followed instructions when taking the drug treatment, and when she later miscarried all eight foetuses. Several questions were raised by the case, not least over the desirability of any woman facing the risks of a multiple pregnancy and birth. Multiple pregnancy is an inevitable risk when women are prescribed superovulatory drugs and the normal risks of pregnancy, such as anaemia and eclampsia, are exacerbated by the sheer mechanical effects of carrying an abdomen full of eight babies Yet in some ways the case was not new. In 1984 Jan and Graham Walton had sextuplet daughters following infertility treatment. As recently as 1993, Jean Vince gave birth to five girls and a boy after refusing a selective abortion.

Meanwhile, Diane Blood is portrayed as the devoted wife who has been sadly wronged by the HFEA.

Briefly, a sperm donation was taken from Diane Blood's husband, Stephen, while he was in a coma as a result of meningitis from which he never recovered, but the authorities refused to let Mrs Blood be inseminated because Stephen had never actively consented to this, despite his wife's belief that post-mortem conception is what he would have wanted. The couple had planned to have a baby and at one point Mrs Blood had thought she was pregnant. The problem hinges on the fact that the Human Fertilisation and Embryology Act of 1990 requires that a man's consent to the use of his sperm must be in writing. Diane Blood's argument is that her husband couldn't so consent because he was unconscious, but that they were actively trying for a baby. If Mrs Blood wanted to be inseminated by an unknown man who had given written consent for his sperm to be used, there would appear to be no problem. As ever, the legalities and the moralities don't necessarily agree. Professor Lord Robert Winston has argued that the case should be taken on its individual merits rather than on a general principle. Another argument is that some laws are needed to govern such treatments.

A test case if ever there was one, Diane Blood's argument was heard by the High Court in October 1996, where permission to use her dead husband's sperm was refused. The British Medical Association's Ethics Committee also turned down her application at that time. She later appealed against the High Court ruling and was granted consent to use the sperm outside the UK. Mrs Blood has since sought treatment in Belgium, which does not have such strict rules.

An article by Bridgit Diamond outlines the legal issues involved.[1] Consent to the use of gametes or embryos has to be given in writing. It is of some consolation, perhaps, to parents of frozen embryos fearing a 'brave new world' that an embryo taken from a woman must not be used for any purpose unless there is an effective consent by her to the use of the embryo for that purpose. Consent may also be withdrawn at any time.

Selective termination

One issue under discussion is that of selective termination or selective reduction. This may occur when several embryos are returned to the uterus after IVF (as replacing more embryos than is strictly necessary may improve the chances of pregnancy occurring) and the woman is later found to be carrying more than twins or triplets. Multiple pregnancies are then reduced by injecting 'excess' foetuses with potassium cyanide to induce selective miscarriage. Such reduction is distasteful to many people, doctors included, and many will remember Mandy Allwood's decision not to terminate any of her multiple embryos despite the risk of losing them all, because such 'culling' is a terrible human predicament.

The welfare of the child

In information provided by the HFEA, one restriction on patients treated relates to 'the welfare of the child. Before offering treatment, clinics must take into account the welfare of the child and the commitment of the people seeking treatment to not only having but also raising a child.' How can this be measured? The booklet suggests that criteria should include: the age and medical histories of families, the risk of harm (such as neglect or abuse) and the effect of a new baby upon any existing children. This is an aspect we hear little about, which has raised justified criticism.

Should infertility be treated on the NHS?

IVF is an expensive solution against which it is easy to take a theoretical stance if you are not infertile. However, there are very real problems of complaints about the lack of services and the difficulties in receiving sympathetic help. Universal IVF provision, if we are to have any at all, should be a major priority, and unequal access to infertility treatment is part of the NHS's failure to meet women's needs generally.

It is hard to assess the effectiveness of infertility services, because of the lack of information. Estimates vary, but one in ten couples are affected at some time – this is 50,000 new cases of infertility each year: probably an underestimate. One in six are thought to need help due to infertility and a two-and-a-half-year wait for such help is average. The NHS pays a lack of attention to infertility – there is no consistent policy, with services patchy and some districts severely under-resourced. The north–south divide is apparent, with the north worse off in terms of provision. If you can afford it, you may still have to travel long distances for private treatment. Some areas simply offer less effective treatment, not updated as it should be, because of fewer facilities – not all, for example, will offer ovarian scanning, microsurgery or radio immune assay services for testing hormone levels. This discriminates against the infertile on low incomes who are often driven (impossibly) to the private sector. There is a lack of commitment in the NHS to the right to have – or not to have – a child. Some people may be excluded for social reasons (for example, lesbians and single heterosexuals may have problems getting artificial insemination on the NHS), so there is some degree of assessment of suitability as parents.

Most IVF treatment is therefore taking place in private clinics in return for fees. Costs vary and medical and travel bills are expensive. It is a service only for the relatively affluent. Some private health insurers don't include such treatments in their policies.

There is a dearth of written or verbal information about the causes of infertility. Likewise, there is an absence of truly valuable counselling. Concentration is on the body, not the mind or spirit. Perhaps it is about time women were encouraged not to believe that motherhood is the single most fulfilling aspect of their lives – indeed, most mothers speaking honestly would probably accept that it isn't.

There should be more research into causes and more information should be given to the young through sex education and general studies. For example, pelvic inflammatory disease is significant as a cause of infertility, but there appears to be little research into PID; this is also true of chlamydia, for which there are few facilities for screening or treatment. The IUD (coil) has been linked with pelvic infection – perhaps more research is needed into this potentially dangerous form of contraception. Women generally need a better health service – gynaecology waiting lists are long. The starting point as far as infertility is concerned is that at the very least the same service should be available free on the NHS.

Is the debate about IVF actually a red herring, diverting attention from the problem of how to prevent infertility in the first place, which there seems little interest in? Why do we tolerate so much dysfunction? Smoking reduces fertility, so why are we not trumpeting the fact and investigating environmental issues while promoting health, not accepting and treating sickness?

As we move forwards into a new millennium, the issues are becoming ever more intense. The battle is between the right of a woman to reproduce versus the ability of the state to provide the necessary resources. As technology and the advance of medicine make miracles a more everyday occurrence, the frustration at being refused access to them is all the greater.

Note

1. Bridgit Diamond, 'In Vitro Fertilisation and the Law' in *Modern Midwife*, vol. 4, no. 12, December 1994, pp. 32–4.

8 If you are seeking treatment

Current guidelines are that you should be actively trying for a baby for at least a year before seeking help, but for some couples the time factor is important, perhaps because of maternal age. The first port of call is usually your GP, who may be able to offer some of the more basic tests and drugs. It is helpful if both partners visit the GP together, as infertility is a joint problem regardless of the cause. Some GPs are unable or unwilling to treat patients for infertility on the NHS – the option is then open to change GP. Unfortunately each district health authority has its own criteria to determine who, if anyone, it will fund. Your community health council (see telephone directory) should be able to tell you what the criteria are in your district. Most clinics will offer private treatment to those who can afford it, but the costs vary widely and it is worth investigating these thoroughly before you begin, especially as budgets can become increasingly stretched the further into infertility treatment you need to go. Check whether charges are all-inclusive or whether drugs are charged separately. Private clinics may also have criteria for people they will not treat, such as single women, so although infertility is an emotional issue, you really need first to go into the investigations with a view to cost and availability to avoid early disappointment.

There are a number of clinics (around 100) spread throughout the UK, so most people will live within a reasonable distance of one. All are regulated by the HFEA. All of these clinics will supply you with written information before offering any treatment and it is certainly worth obtaining and reading this. The HFEA has a Patients' Guide which will answer many of your questions about clinics' comparative costs/treatments in statistical form. You are fully entitled to visit the clinics and see the staff before making a decision, especially if you are opting for private treatment.

Not all infertility requires such advanced techniques as IVF. Many people can be treated with drug therapy by their GP, or may have damaged fallopian tubes assessed or cleared at their local hospital's gynaecology department.

You need to check waiting lists for various treatments. Be warned – these are generally long. If your procedure will involve donated eggs, you are probably in for the longest wait of all: not only are they in short supply but they need to be matched so that donor and recipient are similar. As with many things in life, it is always worth chasing up treatment and not relying on bureaucratic systems to keep you informed.

Incidentally, advice from the association CHILD is that you should not wait as long as a year before seeking treatment for infertility if:

1. The woman is over 35 years of age.
2. She has absent or irregular periods.
3. She has had abdominal or pelvic surgery.
4. The man has had surgery to the groin or injury to the testicles.
5. Either partner has ever had a sexually transmitted disease.
6. There is a possible genetic reason.

Useful addresses

BAAF (British Agencies for Adoption and Fostering)
Skyline House, 200 Union Street, London SEI OLX
Tel: 0171 593 2000
Organisation concerned with adoption and fostering arrangements

CHILD
Charter House, 43, St Leonard's Road, Bexhill on Sea, East Sussex TN40 1JA
Tel: 01424 732361
Self-help organisation for those suffering from infertility.

COTS (Childlessness Overcome through Surrogacy)
Loandhu Cottage, Gruids, Lairg, Sutherland, Scotland IV27 4EF
Tel: 01549 402401
Organisation that seeks to put couples in touch with potential surrogate mothers.

Cromwell IVF Centres
Located at Cromwell Hospital, London, the Sunderland NHS Trust, Swansea Hospital and Washington Hospital. Pioneering centres for egg sharing.

DI Network
PO Box 265, Sheffield S3 7YX
Tel: 0181 245 4369
A national association covering the issues associated with donor insemination and egg donation.

The Family Planning Association
27 Mortimer Street,
London W1N 7RJ
Tel: 0171 636 7866
Advises on contraception, infertility and psychosexual counselling throughout Britain.

Foresight (Association for the Promotion of Preconceptul Care)
28 The Paddock, Godalming, Surrey GU7 1XD
Tel: 01483 427839
Advises on the achievement of optimum health before conception.

HFEA (Human Fertility and Embryology Authority)
Paxton House, 30 Artillery Lane, London E1 7LS
Tel: 0171 377 5077
The regulatory authority for clinics providing IVF and related treatments.

IFIPA (International Federation of Infertility Patients' Associations)
BP2, 78 670 Villennes-sur-Seine, France
Tel: 00 33 1 39 75 66 42
A combined forum for infertility associations throughout the world.

Impotence Association
PO Box 10296, London SW17 7ZN

Impotence Information Centre
PO Box 1130, London W3 OBB
Aims to support medical practitioners, the public and the media with news about recent developments in the treatment of male sexual dysfunction.

ISSUE
509 Aldridge Road, Great Barr, Birmingham B44 8NA
Tel: 0121 344 4414
A patient support group also offering information and representation to those with fertility problems.

NCT Special Experiences Register
Tel: (9–12 noon) Barbara Reynolds 0181 992 8637; (1–8pm) Fiona Hird 0191 415 1857
Tries to provide a personal link with someone who has experienced similar problems.

NEEDS (National Egg and Embryo Donation Society)
Tel: 0161 276 6000
Provides information for potential egg donors.

NIAC (National Infertility Awareness Campaign)
PO Box 2106, London WIA 3D2
Tel: 0800 716 345 (free phone)
The campaigning and lobbying arm of infertility sufferers.

TAMBA (Twins and Multiple Births Association)
PO Box 30, Little Sutton, South Wirral, Merseyside L66 ITH
Tel: 0151 348 0020
Offers help and support to parents of twins, triplets, quads and so on.

Tavistock Marital Studies Institute
120 Belsize Lane, London NW3 5BA
Tel: 0171 435 7111
Consultation service for couples experiencing difficulties in their relationship arising from infertility.

Postscript

If the last twenty years since the birth of Louise Brown have been a period of consolidation and innovation – improving treatments and making them more accessible to thousands of would-be parents – the next twenty years should be equally ground-breaking but the questions surrounding infertility and its treatment will not go away.

There have been some marvellous breakthroughs in treatment but there a number of ethical issues which remain problematic. After the completion of this book, Dr Paul Rainsbury started the first sex selection fertility programme in the UK, a move which has attracted a hostile reaction not unlike that first received by Steptoe and Edwards. The criticisms are easy to deduce and understandable, but on a worldwide scale where sex selection in many countries is currently practised after birth, with millions of babies condemned to infanticide, the issue is by no means clear cut. There may be benefits to sex selection in some cases, but such engineering, if practised on a wide scale, would be bound to have social repercussions.

A report in the *Sunday Times* (9 November, 1997) noted that scientists have found a way of providing lifelong fertility whereby women could delay childbirth until they were in their fifties or even later. This procedure involves a chemical implant that women can have in their early twenties and ensures the maximum preservation of egg stores. The therapy is still at the experimental trial stage in the USA, but many are already worried about having 70- or 80-year-old mothers still responsible for their children. At the same time the age at which men become natural fathers is rarely questioned; indeed, fathers of pensionable age are applauded as 'laddish' rather than irresponsible.

Despite improvements in live birth success rates for fertility treatments, there remain technical problems. Additionally, as new techniques develop, the downside invariable comes to light.

A 1997 study has discovered that infants conceived by ICSI are more than twice as likely to have serious birth defects and nearly 50 per cent more likely to have a minor defect.[1] The study has revealed cardiovascular, genito-urinary and gastrointestinal defects, plus there are cleft palate and diaphragmatic hernia problems. Under normal circumstances, such sperm would probably not produce a pregnancy at all. Manipulation may not always have ideal results and couples opting for ICSI need to be aware of the potential risks.

Sperm seems to be the hot topic in the infertility debate for future years. As this book goes to press, the HFEA is warning of a growing trade offering the services of potential sperm donors on the world wide web. Several agencies have already sprung up, offering donated sperm for around £280 ($450) per sample. Detailed profiles of donors cost a little more. It was bound to happen but is again fraught with difficulties – the HFEA warns of the potential for contracting diseases such as syphilis, HIV or hepatitis from unscreened sperm. Additionally, such sperm may be of poor quality with recipients doomed to disappointment when it fails to fertilise. Sadly, the desperation to reproduce means that the unscrupulous have a handy means of making cash at their disposal by exploiting the vulnerable.[2]

The mid-1990s have produced some spectacular headlines on the issue of fertility treatment. Sadly, the tabloid newspapers thrive on stories about selective abortion, cloning, the sale of eggs, surrogacy, destruction of embryos, and the cost of HIV patients receiving IVF. On the other hand the recent spate of articles and TV programmes have brought the issues surrounding infertility out of the closet and have played a role in removing some of the stigma attached to infertility. The reality is that most parents undergoing infertility treatment are not undertaking processes, like IVF, lightly. They are people suffering the emotional and social consequences of being childless in a family orientated society.

The financial aspect of fertility treatment remains (for the foreseeable future) a controversial one. A 1997 survey has shown that an estimated 90 per cent of babies born by IVF are conceived in private treatment and 19 per cent of health authorities (who responded to the survey) do not purchase IVF.[3] The lottery remains. But the public purse is finite; two cycles of GIFT or IVF to 50 couples per annum costs around £140,000 and the multiple births add extra neonatal costs. And the patchy provision of treatment continues. Wendy and Richard, whose story is told in this book, have learnt that their three year wait for NHS IVF has been extended, for no apparent reason, to four years. Other couples question the advice given by medical professionals. Cheryl and Andrew were told there was no chance of natural conception occurring. After three failed IVF attempts, they are now proud parents of a naturally conceived daughter, Amy. Numerous couples, finding no reason for their infertility are almost automatically referred for IVF without full and proper investigations – a costly process and traumatic for the people concerned.

Childless couples don't always receive the information, advice and support that they need; partly because the causes of infertility are still not clearly understood. In a society which loves babies (but, some would argue, not children) little help is given to people who decide to remain childless. Those who might consider adoption are told to choose between fertility treatment and adoption, neither of which may work. Since the birth of Louise Brown, we have indeed witnessed great breakthroughs in IVF treatment but we also need changes in societal attitudes, to tackle the ethical decisions that lag behind the technology, and to pay more than lip-service to the plight of the infertile.

Notes

1. Kurinczuk, J.J. and Bower, C., 'Birth Defects in Infants Conceived by Intracytoplasmic Sperm Injection: An Alternative Interpretation', *British Medical Journal*, vol. 315, 1997, pp. 1260–1266.
2. Mihill, Chris, 'Infertile couples told not to buy "unchecked" sperm via Internet', *Guardian*, 28 January, 1998.
3. 'Do We Have a Right to Reproduce?', *Nursing Times*, September 3–9, 1997.

Glossary

Abortion
The premature expulsion of an embryo from the uterus. When an abortion is deliberate, it is known as an induced abortion, voluntary abortion, therapeutic abortion, or termination of pregnancy. When it occurs naturally, it is known as a spontaneous abortion or miscarriage.

Adhesion
A band of scar tissue that binds organs together; most likely to form after infection or operation.

AID
Artificial insemination by donor's sperm.

AIH
Artificial insemination by husband's (or partner's) sperm.

Amniocentesis
Removal of a small sample of amniotic fluid from the uterus during pregnancy for chromosome analysis, to determine potential foetal defects.

Antibody
A substance produced in the body that attacks foreign bacteria or viruses. It is possible for both men and women to produce antibodies against sperm, which can cause infertility.

Artificial insemination
Injection of semen by syringe into a woman's cervix. If a husband's/partner's semen is used, it is known as AIH; if a donor's semen is used, it is AID.

Azoospermia
Complete absence of sperm in semen.

Benign tumour
A tumour that grows slowly but does not invade surrounding tissue. Benign tumours are not dangerous.

Buserilin
A hormone suppressant given by nasal spray or daily injection. It suppresses the action of the pituitary gland, which normally stimulates the ovaries to produce eggs.

Caesarean section
Delivery of a child through an incision in the abdominal wall rather than through the vagina.

Cervical mucus
The secretions surrounding the cervical canal. The amount and texture change during ovulation to allow sperm penetration.

Cervix
The neck of the uterus, opening into the vagina.

Chlamydia
A micro-organism found in the genito-urinary tract; often transmitted via sexual contact.

Chorionic villi sampling
A test performed early in pregnancy as an indicator of foetal defects.

Clomid
Brand name for the non-steroid oestrogen clomiphene citrate, a fertility drug used to stimulate ovaries.

Cloning
The production of an organism, asexually, from a single ancestor.

Conceptus
A fertilised ovum or, later, the embryo, foetus, placenta and other membranes.

Corpus luteum
The 'yellow body' which develops in the ovarian follicle after an ovum has been produced. It secretes progesterone.

Cryopreservation
Preservation of tissue by freezing.

Culture
A laboratory procedure in which organisms (in this case particularly human ova) are encouraged to develop.

Cyclogest
A drug, available on prescription, used to control female hormone levels to maintain a pregnancy in its very early stage.

D&C (dilatation and curettage)
A minor surgical procedure in which the cervix is dilated to permit scraping of the uterine wall with an instrument called a curette.

Danazol
A drug used to treat endometriosis, marketed under the brand name Danol.

Echovist
A new technique, an ultrasound procedure very similar to a hysterosalpingogram but without the need for X-rays.

Eclampsia
A fairly rare, serious condition of late pregnancy, labour and delivery, believed to be caused by excess fluid swelling in the woman's brain.

Ectopic pregnancy
A dangerous condition in which a fertilised ovum attaches itself outside the uterus (usually in a fallopian tube) and begins to grow.

Egg
Female sex cell, female gamete, ovum.

Embryo
An early stage of prenatal development, to the eighth week of pregnancy. Beyond this time, the term foetus is applied.

Endometriosis
A condition characterised by abnormal growth of endometrial cells in areas of the pelvis outside the uterus.

Endometrium
The mucus membrane that lines the uterus.

Eugenics
Research aimed at producing healthy offspring and thus 'perfecting' the human race. Usually associated with intolerance of any disability or learning difficulty.

Fallopian tube
The long, narrow tube between an ovary and the uterus. After release of the egg from the ovary, the tube transports the egg to the uterus.

Fertilisation
Penetration of ovum by sperm.

Fertility
The ability to produce offspring; a woman's ability to conceive and carry a child or a man's ability to impregnate a woman.

Fertility drugs
Drugs that stimulate an ovary to release an ovum.

Foetus
An unborn conceptus after eight weeks in the uterus.

Folic acid
A vitamin of the B group, a deficiency of which is known to be a potential contributory factor in an unborn child's developing spina bifida. Women considering pregnancy are urged to supplement their folic acid.

Follicle
A small sac in the ovary in which the ovum develops.

Follicle-stimulating hormone (FSH)
A hormone produced by the pituitary gland. In women it is secreted cyclically and is responsible for ripening the egg. In men it is essential for sperm growth.

Gametes
A male sperm cell or female egg cell (ovum).

Genetic engineering
The deliberate manipulation of hereditary features by treatment to transfer particular genes.

GIFT (gamete intrafallopian transfer)
A fertility assistance procedure. Eggs are collected from the ovary and returned to the fallopian tubes, along with a sperm sample, for fertilisation to take place as naturally as possible.

GNRH argonist
A drug which prevents the working of the female body's normal ovulatory controls.

Gonadotrophins
Pituitary hormones that stimulate the reproduction system.

Gynaecologist
A specialist in the care of the female reproductive system.

Heperin
A drug, administered intravenously by medical professionals, which prevents blood clotting.

Hormone
A chemical secreted by the endocrine glands that circulates in the blood to regulate many body functions. Hormones are also made synthetically.

Human chorionic gonadotrophin (HCG)
A hormone secreted by the placenta during pregnancy. Its presence in the blood indicates a positive pregnancy test. It may be used with other hormones in treating infertility.

Human menopausal gonadotrophin (HMG)
Extracted from the urine of post-menopausal women, this contains FSH. It is used in the treatment of fertility problems.

Humegon
One of a group of drugs that emulate the action of hormones to promote the production of eggs within the body.

Hypothalamus
The primitive lower region of the brain.

Hysterectomy
Surgical removal of the uterus.

Hysterosalpingogram (HSG)
An X-ray study performed by injecting dye into the uterus to examine the interior of the uterus and fallopian tubes.

ICSI (intracytoplasmic sperm injection)
A form of assisted conception, whereby a single sperm is injected into an egg. If it fertilises, it is transferred to the uterus.

Implantation
The process by which the fertilised ovum attaches itself to the endometrium.

Impotence
Inability of the male to produce or maintain an erection.

Infertility
Inability to produce offspring. May be permanent or may refer to a prolonged, temporary status.

Insemination
The impregnation of an ovum by a sperm.

Internal pelvic examination
A physical examination in which the physician feels the shape of the internal reproductive organs of the female by inserting two

fingers into the vagina while pressing down on the abdomen with the other hand. Also called bimanual examination.

Intrauterine
Within the uterus.

Intrauterine device (IUD)
A contraceptive device, inserted into the uterus to prevent pregnancy.

In vitro fertilisation (IVF)
Fertilisation that takes place outside the body. Also called extracorporeal fertilisation.

IUI (interuterine insemination)
A form of assisted conception, whereby ova are stimulated with the aid of drugs and inseminated inside the uterus with the use of a catheter and sperm sample.

Laparascope
A telescopic instrument inserted through a small incision in the navel to examine the pelvic cavity.

Laparoscopy
Examination with a laparascope.

Laparotomy
A major surgical procedure in which the abdomen is opened through incision in the abdominal wall.

LH
See Luteinising hormone.

LH-RH
Releasing hormone from the hypothalamus which activates FSH and LH in men and women.

Luteinising hormone (LH)
A hormone secreted by the pituitary gland. In women, it is produced cyclically to stimulate the body to manufacture progesterone. In men, it stimulates testicular cells to produce testosterone.

Lymphoma
A malignant tumour that forms in a lymph gland.

MESA (Microsurgical epidydimal sperm aspiration)
A form of ICSI treatment in which a single immature sperm can be used to inseminate an egg.

Metrodin
A more recent version of Perganol, one of a group of drugs used to control female hormone levels.

Miscarriage
Spontaneous loss of the foetus or embryo from the womb.

Motility
Ability to move, in particular the movement of sperm within the seminal fluid.

Nafarelin
A GNRH drug, available on prescription and taken via a nasal spray.

Normegon
One of a group of drugs that emulate the action of hormones to promote the production of eggs within the body.

Obstetrician
A specialist in the care of pregnant women.

Oestrogen
A major female sex hormone, secreted mainly by the ovaries in women and in smaller amounts by the adrenals in men and women.

Oral contraceptive
A substance (such as the birth control pill) taken by mouth to prevent pregnancy.

Orgaful
One of a group of drugs that emulate the action of hormones to promote the production of eggs within the body.

Ovarian hyperstimulation syndrome
A possible side effect of fertility treatment. The ovaries react to drugs by overproducing follicles, endangering the health of the woman and the quality of the ova.

Ovary
One of a pair of female glands, located on either side of the uterus (to which they are connected by the fallopian tubes). Egg cells develop in follicles in the ovaries, which also produce oestrogen and progesterone.

Ovulatim
The production of an ovum from the ovary, usually on a regular, cyclical basis.

Ovum
The female egg cell.

Patency
Openness, as of the fallopian tubes.

Pelvic inflammatory disease (PID)
Generalised infection of the female reproductive organs.

Pergonal
Brand name for a mixture of 50 per cent luteinising hormone and 50 per cent follicle-stimulating hormone, extracted from postmenopausal female urine. A potent ovulation-induction drug, it has been known to produce multiple pregnancies.

Peritoneum
The tissue covering the inside of the abdomen wall.

Peritonitis
Inflammation of the peritoneum.

Pethidene
A painkilling drug, administered by medical professionals.

Pituitary gland
A gland located at the base of the brain that is responsible for many hormone secretions in the body.

Placenta
A spongy substance in the uterus that links the blood supply of mother and foetus.

Placenta praevia
A condition of some pregnancies in which the placenta is situated very low down in the uterus, blocking the infant's passage into the cervix and so necessitating delivery by Caesarean section.

Polycystic ovarian disease (PCO)
A condition in which the presence of a large number of ovarian cysts prevents fertility.

Post-coital test
Performed 24–36 hours after conception, this test shows whether the cervical mucus in the woman's body is receptive to, and compatible with her partner's sperm.

Premarin
Brand name of a hormonal component of 'conjugated oestrogens' derived from horse oestrogen.

Premature menopause
Menopause occurring when a woman is in her 30s or earlier. The cause is not known.

Primulet N
A drug available on prescription which caused the onset of menstruation.

Profasi
A drug, administered by medical professionals, which prepares human eggs for conception.

Progesterone
The major female hormone secreted by the corpus luteum and other organs during pregnancy.

Prolactin
A hormone released by a woman's pituitary gland.

Prostaglandins
Hormones in the blood that have an effect on metabolism and blood vessels and that cause the mouth muscle to either contract or relax. It is carried through the body in prostatic fluid.

Prostap
A GNRH drug, available on prescription and taken via a subcutaneous injection.

Radio immune assay services
A modern, non-invasive method of testing human hormone levels.

Secondary infertility
Infertility in a couple who have already had one or more successful pregnancies. Sometimes called one-child sterility.

Semen
The milky fluid of the ejaculate, comprised of sperm and secretions.

Semen analysis
Laboratory study of semen under the microscope to examine the number, size, shape and motility of sperm.

Sonohysterogram
Non-invasive examination of the uterus and fallopian tubes, performed with the aid of external sound transmission.

Sperm
Short for spermatozoon (pl. spermatozoa): the fully developed male reproductive cell.

Sperm count
A laboratory examination to count the number and characteristics of sperm in the ejaculate.

Sperm wash
A technique whereby a sperm sample is diluted with culture medium and then suspended in fresh culture medium, allowing the best quality sperm to swim up to the top layer of the medium and so be harvested for insemination.

Stemetil
A drug, administered by medical professionals, which controls nausea and vomiting.

Sterile
Permanently infertile.

Sterilisation
A procedure that terminates fertility by interrupting the male or female reproductive system.

Subfertility
A delay in producing offspring due to some problem in conception.

Surrogacy
Replacement of one person by a deputy – in this context, the use of a substitute who will carry a child for another woman.

SUZI (sub-zonal insemination)
A procedure, commonly used in assisting fertility, whereby a single sperm is injected into an egg and the egg replaced within the prospective mother's body.

Synoral
A drug, available on prescription, which removes the body's ability to ovulate.

Temperature chart
The chart kept by a woman of her daily body temperature to determine when or if she ovulates.

TESE (testicular sperm extraction)
A form of ICSI treatment in which a single immature sperm can be used to inseminate an egg.

Test-tube baby
Popular term for a child produced by fertilisation outside the body.

Testis (pl. testes)
One of the two male sex organs, or testicles, which produce sperm.

Ultrasonography (ultrasound)
A diagnostic technique that uses sound waves, rather than X-rays, to visualise internal body structures.

Uterine
Pertaining to the uterus.

Uterus
The womb: a hollow, muscular organ in the woman where the foetus develops.

Vagina
The birth canal; the passage between cervix and vulva.

Venereal disease
Any disease transmitted by sexual intercourse.

ZIFT (zygote intrafallopian transfer)
A fertility assistance procedure, whereby eggs are stimulated, collected, fertilised and returned directly to the fallopian tubes.

Zoladex
A GNRH drug, available on prescription and taken via a subcutaneous injection.

Bibliography and helpful reading

Bibliography

Biggs, Sarah and Ironside, Virginia, *The Subfertility Handbook*, Sheldon Press, 1995

Brewer, Sarah, *Endometriosis and Fibroids*, Vermilion, 1997

Connors Steve, 'Male Infertility Linked to Birth Defect', Foresight spring newsletter, February 1997

HFEA, *The Patients' Guide to DI and IVF Clinics* (free of charge: tel: 0171 377 5077)

King's ACU Support Group, *The Infertility Patients' Directory* (tel: 0171 274 3242)

McTaggart, Lynne, *What Doctors Don't Tell You*, vol. 7, no. 7, October, 1996

Malone, Chris, 'Managing Multiple Births. Part 1: The Quest for Parenthood', in *Modern Midwife*, vol. 5, no. 9, September 1995

Helpful reading

Fiction:
Asher, Jane, *The Longing: A Novel*, Harper Collins, 1996

Maitland, Sarah, *Daughter of Jerusalem*, Virago, 1993

Non-fiction:
Badinter, Elizabeth, *The Myth of Motherhood*, Souvenir, 1982

Bradley, Suzanne Gail and Bennett, Nicholas, *Preparation for Pregnancy: An Essential Guide*, Argyll Publishing, 1995

Cargreaves, Kate, *Journey to our Children*, Aurora Publishing, 1996

Coburn, Theo, Myers, John Peterson, and Dumanski, Dianne, *Our Stolen Future*, Little, Brown, 1996

Diamond, Bridgit, 'In Vitro Fertilisation and the Law', in *Modern Midwife*, vol. 4, no. 12, December 1994, pp. 32–4.

Eck Manning, Barbara, *Infertility*, Simon & Schuster, 1987

Furse, Anna, *The Infertility Companion: A Users Guide to Tests, Technologies and Therapies*, Thorsons, 1997

Hampshire, Susan, *The Maternal Instinct*, Sidgwick, 1984

Jones, Maggie, *Infertility: Modern Treatments and the Issues They Raise*, Piatkus, 1991

Klein, Renate D., *Infertility: Women Speak Out*, Pandora, 1989

Snowdon, Elizabeth and Robert, *The Gift of a Child*, University of Exeter Press, 1993

Stanworth, Michelle (ed.), *Reproductive Technologies: Gender, Motherhood and Medicine*, Polity Press, 1987

Steptoe, Patrick and Edwards, Robert, *A Matter of Life*, Hutchinson, 1980

Stonehouse, Julia, *Idols and Incubators*, Scarlet Press 1994

Thurer, Shari L., *The Myths of Motherhood: How Culture Reinvents the Good Mother*, Penguin, 1995

Wesson, Nicky, *Alternative Treatments for Infertility*, Vermillion, 1997

Winston, Professor Robert, *Infertility: A Sympathetic Approach*, Optima, 1993

Winston, Professor Robert, *Making Babies: A Personal View of IVF Treatment*, BBC, 1996

Index

Also by Jo Benson and Dawn Robinson-Walsh

Love, Labour and Loss
Stillbirth and Neonatal Death

For many parents the loss of a child through neonatal death or stillbirth is often their first close encounter with bereavement. With personal testimony from many who have experienced loss, this book gives positive and practical help.

'This book is a deeply moving tribute to the babies who have known so short a life and who have left a significant impact on the people who loved and longed for them. These parents are now helping others to better understand the feelings involved in grief and loss.' Jenni Thomas, Director, the Child Bereavement Trust

'*Love, Labour and Loss* is something bereaved parents will welcome as it so clearly expresses many of the feelings that they have had or will have in the future ... For newly bereaved parents it will offer them some comfort that they are not alone in their feelings, that other people have been there too.' Stillbirth and Neonatal Death Society (SANDS)

ISBN 1 85727 063 0